Know the Early Warning Signs of a Problem Prostate!

- fever and chills
- any difficulty urinating
- pain in the lower back, muscles, or joints
- tender or swollen prostate
- painful ejaculation
- pain in the perineum
  (the area between the scrotum and anus)

In recent years, medical science has made tremendous progress in the detection and treatment of prostate disorders. But your own participation in your prostate health care can be just as vital as the assistance of expert physicians and researchers. THE PROSTATE ANSWER BOOK can help you choose the right doctor and make informed decisions should the occasion arise—and most of all, help prevent serious problems from happening in the first place.

THE PROSTATE ANSWER BOOK

THE PROSTATE ANSWER BOOK

All the causes, all the treatments
for one of the most serious problems
facing men today

Roberta Altman

WARNER BOOKS

A Time Warner Company

WARNER BOOKS EDITION

Cover design by Julia Kushnirsky

Warner Books, Inc.
1271 Avenue of the Americas
New York, NY 10020

 A Time Warner Company

Printed in the United States of America

First Printing: December, 1993

10 9 8 7 6 5 4 3 2 1

DEDICATION

To my father, Martin K. Altman, who died before his time of prostate cancer, and my dear friend Les, who was diagnosed early enough to be treated and cured.

ACKNOWLEDGMENTS

Many people took time out from busy days to assist me in making this book as current and comprehensive as possible. Special thanks go to urologist Michael Solomon, M.D., at the Robert Woods Johnson Hospital in New Jersey. Thanks as well to Patrick Walsh, M.D., at Johns Hopkins Medical Institute in Baltimore; Joel Karp, M.D., F.A.C.S., at Maimonides Medical Center in Brooklyn, New York; clinical psychologist Ursula Ofman, Ph.D.; Karrie Zampini, A.C.S.W., director of the Post-Treatment Resource Center at the Memorial Sloan-Kettering Cancer Center; Joanne Frankel, R.N.; and Randy Jacobs, R.N.

Thank you to the many patients who generously shared with me their experience with prostate disease.

Many of the organizations listed in the book were also helpful, including the American Cancer Society, the National Cancer Institute, and the American Foundation for Urologic Disease.

Last but certainly not least are my editor at Warner Books, Joann Davis, whose comments and suggestions strengthened this book; and Janis Vallely, my agent, who was always there and even sent clippings!

TABLE OF CONTENTS

FOREWORD

As the male population ages, the likelihood of being affected by prostate disease escalates substantially. Prostate cancer is now the most common cancer in men. One in eleven men in the United States will be diagnosed with prostate cancer during his lifetime. After lung cancer, prostate cancer is the leading cause of cancer death in men. The incidence of prostate cancer rose 47% from 1973 to 1987. Surgery for benign prostatic hypertrophy is the most common operation performed in elderly men.

Substantial progress has been made in our understanding, diagnosis, and treatment of these diseases. Prostate cancer has gotten more exposure in the media than ever before. Though public awareness and patient education are also growing, the pace is much slower. There are still many men who have no idea, or wrong ideas, on what the different diseases of the prostate are, how they can be affected by them, and what the alternative forms of treatment are.

Once confronted with a diagnosis, many patients and family members face fear, anxiety, uncertainty, and confusion. Physicians make an effort to address these problems, but all too often, patients find this inadequate for a variety of reasons. When they hear the diagnosis of cancer they are so shocked that, under great stress, they virtually hear nothing that follows. Or they are confused and don't know what questions to ask. Or they ask the questions and don't understand the answers.

The Prostate Answer Book is a timely resource for patients and their families. It contains the most up to date information about detection, diagnostic tests, treatment and side effects in a style more suitable for the usual patient than the medical terminology provided by many physicians.

One of the more difficult challenges facing patients today is understanding the growing number of options for treating prostate diseases. Patients can no longer be presented with a single recommendation for treating benign prostatic hypertrophy or prostate cancer because the number of treatments available has grown considerably. For example, in early stage prostate cancer the treatment may be surgery (removing the tumor), radiation therapy, or expectant treatment which is no initial treatment but regular followup and treatment when and if symptoms occur.

Making a selection on which treatment to choose is a balance between the relative advantages and disadvantages. That is often confusing when discussed solely in the physician's office. The patient understandably is concerned about making the best decision on which treatment to undergo. Something else is definitely needed. *The Prostate Answer Book* fills that need. It can serve as a helpful supplement to the information supplied by the physician. The patient can use the information in the book to review the various treatment options mentioned by his doctor—their risks, side effects, advantages and disadvantages, how they're performed—before making his decision. It will enhance his ability to evaluate the various options open to him and facilitate his understanding. It also provides an easy way to make information about the disease and its treatment accessible to anxious family members who were not in the doctors office and want very much to understand what is happening so they can be supportive.

When this information is combined with the medical information provided by their doctor, patients should have greater awareness and feel more comfortable participating in the decision-making process to select the most appropriate treatment. This can be helpful to the physician as well. When the patient and his family know and understand what is happening, the physician's job is easier and the patient and family members are likely to feel more positive about their experience.

Finally, *The Prostate Answer Book* discusses other organizations which can give additional information and support to patients. One in particular, of which I am very aware, is called US TOO, which every man with prostate cancer should know about. US TOO is a national support group for prostate cancer patients and their families. It was founded in 1990 by a patient at the University of Chicago who wanted to talk with other men going through what he was going through. Now there are groups all over the country.

I believe that this book can be immeasurably helpful to patients and family members; and make a tough and often frightening experience a little easier to get through.

Gerald W. Chodak, M.D., F.A.C.S.
Professor of Surgery/Urology
Director of Prostate and Urology Center
The University of Chicago

NOTE TO THE READER

Because *The Prostate Answer Book* is written for the layperson, it is designed to be as easy to use and understand as possible. Since there may be people who will not read this book from cover to cover—and may head directly to the section which concerns them—I have occasionally repeated some information that I think is important and not to be missed. For example, there are several references to the guidelines for the digital rectal examination (DRE), which can detect prostate cancer very early, when it is most curable. Also, I frequently repeat, in parentheses, abbreviations of a procedure so that it is not necessary to thumb back in the text as you think, "I know I saw the letters TURP some pages ago . . . but what is it?"

In medical language, as in all language, there can be two or three names for the same thing. That can be very confusing, especially when it is terminology with which you are not familiar. When more than one name or term is used for the same thing, the other names are indicated.

A good portion of this book does deal with cancer. That is because prostate cancer is the most serious problem than can affect the prostate and cancer carries with it a lot of other baggage besides the physical disease, such as its emotional impact on the patient and on the family members.

There are practical suggestions for dealing with side effects of the treatment of prostate disease, especially cancer. And there are suggestions on how to deal with the many different emotions engendered by prostate disease.

There is also a fairly extensive glossary of words in the back of the book that you may hear in relation to the prostate. And I have added an appendix of organizations which can provide help in different ways. The kind of assistance they offer is indicated. Whenever there is a toll-free number, it is underlined for easier access. Also included is a bibliography of books offering additional information on the topics in the book.

The Prostate:
What It Is,
Where It Is, and
What It Does

The prostate is one of the male sex glands. It produces the semen, which carries the sperm out of the man's body. In an adult man, a healthy prostate gland is about the size of a walnut. It is located at the base of the penis, right under the bladder, in front of the rectum. It surrounds the first inch or so of the urethra, the tube that runs through the penis and carries semen from the prostate and urine from the bladder to outside the body. It normally has a consistency that is similar to the tip of your nose.

At birth the prostate is minute, about the size of a pea, weighing just a fraction of an ounce. (Even then, it can be felt by a doctor!) It remains relatively small until puberty begins. At that point the prostate enlarges at a much faster pace as a result of stimulation by androgen hormones, substances manufactured in the body which produce male physical characteristics such as facial hair and a deep voice. Weighing in at under an ounce, the prostate stops growing when a man is in his twenties. That's when the prostate is about the size of a walnut. It starts enlarging again when a man is in his forties or fifties. It is rare, but there are some (lucky) men whose prostate gland does not enlarge and actually may decrease in size. It is not really understood why the prostate enlarges and why, in a small percentage of men, it doesn't. However, if you are like most men, your prostate will start growing again when you are forty-five—give or take a few years. This is not at all unusual. And it is not necessarily a problem. However, it is also not unusual for it to eventually become a problem.

The prostate is described as having three zones—central, peripheral, and transitional, made up of some forty tubes (saclike glands) that are lined with mucous membrane. They are surrounded by muscle and elastic fibrous tissue and are contained within a capsule. However, the prostate gland is commonly thought of and referred to by the general public and doctors alike simply as the prostate.

The prostate gland is an accessory or secondary sex gland although, for all practical purposes, its sole function is sexual. It's an "accessory" because it is indirectly involved in reproduction. (The testicles and penis are primary sexual structures because the testicles make the sperm that can fertilize the egg in a woman's body and the penis delivers the sperm.) Normal functioning of the prostate depends on the presence of the male hormone testosterone. The prostate gland, as do all glands, secretes a substance. That substance is semen, a thick, whitish, protein-rich fluid that carries the sperm out of the body. During the male's orgasm the sperm (from the testicles) and semen (from the prostate gland, along with fluid from the seminal vesicles) flood the urethra. The prostate has muscle tissue that squeezes the semen into the urethra. The semen's role is to transport the sperm, which is then ejaculated by the penis. It is believed that the semen

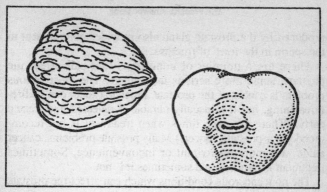

The prostate is about the size of a walnut and consists of a glandular body (saclike gland), muscle and elastic fibrous tissue. (courtesy of *Primary Care & Cancer*)

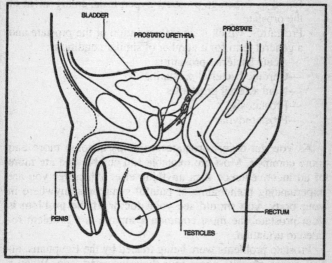

The prostate gland is located at the base of the penis under the bladder and in front of the rectum. (*Prostate Cancer Education Council*)

produced by the prostate gland also provides nourishment to the sperm in the form of fructose.

There are a number of conditions that can affect the prostate, some more serious than others. The most serious problem is cancer of the prostate. Prostate cancer can be life-threatening, but it is usually curable if detected and treated early. (There are even times when treatment is not recommended for prostate cancer!) Many prostate problems, cancer aside, are more an irritant or inconvenience. Sometimes treatment is required and sometimes it is not.

The noncancerous conditions which can affect the prostate are:

- Benign prostatic hypertrophy (BPH), which is also referred to as benign prostatic hyperplasia, enlargement of the prostate
- Prostatitis, which is an inflammation of the prostate and a general term for a number of similar conditions:
  —Acute bacterial prostatitis
  —Chronic bacterial prostatitis
  —Nonbacterial prostatitis
  —Prostatosis
  —Prostatodynia

As you get older, prostate problems become more and more common. Most are treatable and curable and are more of an inconvenience than anything else. Whenever you are experiencing bothersome or painful symptoms anywhere in your body, you should see your doctor. If the problem is your prostate, the most common symptom is a problem related to urination.

Prostate problems were being treated by the Egyptians, albeit rather crudely, some four thousand years ago. When a man was unable to urinate, reeds, copper, or silver tubes would be inserted through the penis and urethra to open the passageway so that the urine could be expelled. It is doubtful that many lives were saved by those early remedies.

The role of the prostate in causing bladder obstruction was first noted in Italy in 1530. In 1649 the first known reference was made to bladder obstruction by a tumor of the prostate. In 1786 a British anatomist showed that by removing the testicles (glands that produce sperm and sex hormones), the growth of the prostate was prevented. He found that when the testicles of mature animals were removed, the prostate atrophied. The first reference to cancer of the prostate was made in 1794. A real understanding of the anatomy and physiology of the prostate did not occur until the early 1900s. In the mid-1930s it was discovered that regression of a prostate tumor could be induced by endocrine (hormonal) manipulation.

There has been tremendous progress in the last half century. *The Prostate Answer Book* examines the controversy surrounding some of the methods of detection and treatment of prostate disease and contains the latest state-of-the-art information on its treatment.

You and
Your Doctor

Your doctor is your first defense against prostate disease through successful treatment. Knowing when to see a doctor, how to choose one, and what to ask is crucial in your ability to maintain good health—of your prostate and your entire body.

WHEN TO GO

Once you turn forty, you should get a digital rectal exam (DRE) every year. The DRE is a simple procedure in which the doctor inserts a gloved, lubricated finger up the rectum. It takes just minutes, is not painful, and is a virtually risk-free procedure. For some men, it is also a dreaded and embarrassing experience, so much so that they simply do not go to the doctor. This is unfortunate, because the DRE enables the doctor to examine your prostate and feel whether it is enlarged or has lumps or other areas of abnormal texture. A

6

DRE, in some cases, can detect prostate cancer in its earliest stage, *before* you experience any symptoms, when it is most likely to be cured. It can also indicate other prostate problems. An annual DRE starting at the age of forty is recommended by the American Cancer Society, the National Cancer Institute, and the American Urological Association. Although there is some controversy about the effectiveness of the DRE, most physicians feel that many lives could be saved if all men followed those guidelines. Naturally, you should not wait a year to see your doctor if you are experiencing symptoms. And you should see a doctor regularly before forty, as well, and whenever you are experiencing symptoms.

Another area of great controversy is the blood test for the prostate-specific antigen (PSA). Elevated levels of this protein in the blood may be an indication of prostate cancer or of benign prostatic disease. Some doctors are now advocating a yearly PSA test as well as a DRE in order to detect prostate cancer when it is present but cannot be detected in a DRE. Other doctors are not convinced that it is practical, cost-effective, or—most important—that it extends survival. (For more information on the PSA, see the chapter on prostate cancer.) In 1992 The American Cancer Society amended its guidelines. It now recommends a yearly PSA test along with the DRE starting at age 50. Although neither a DRE nor PSA is conclusive, they can detect some prostate cancers which have produced no symptoms. If you are 40 or older you should go once a year for a digital rectal exam and go to see your doctor if you have any of the symptoms listed below.

The following symptoms may be an indication of a prostate problem:

- Fever
- Chills
- Any difficulty urinating

- Difficulty in starting to urinate
- A sudden inability to urinate
- More and more frequent urination
- A sense of urgency so that it is hard to postpone urination
- Awakening frequently during the night to urinate
- While urinating, the stream stops and starts
- A sense that your bladder has not been fully emptied
- A bloated abdomen with urine leakage
- Blood in the urine
- A weak urinary stream
- Burning or pain during urination
- Low back pain
- Joint or muscle pain
- Tender or swollen prostate
- Painful ejaculation
- Hematospermia (hemospermia)—slight bleeding with ejaculation (although often a frightening symptom by itself, is seldom a sign of serious illness)
- Pain or discomfort in the perineum, the area between the scrotum and anus

WHOM TO SEE

If you saw your regular doctor and not a urologist (a doctor who specializes in diseases of the urinary tract and sex organs in men), he or she may recommend that you see a urologist if:

- He or she is not sure that you have benign prostatic hypertrophy (BPH), a condition in which the prostate is enlarged
- You do have BPH and the symptoms are bothersome to you
- You are not able to urinate

- You have repeated urinary infections
- There is a suspicion of cancer

Generally your regular doctor can do any preliminary tests, such as the DRE, especially when you are symptom free. You do not necessarily have to see a specialist immediately. However, if you are experiencing symptoms and they are severe, you may save a step by going directly to a urologist.

HOW TO CHOOSE A UROLOGIST

There are a number of ways to choose a urologist. One of the best is word of mouth. Ask a friend which urologist he sees and if he is satisfied with the treatment he has received. You can ask your regular doctor to refer you to a urologist. (If your doctor wants you to see a urologist, he or she will probably give you the name of a urologist to call.) You can call a nearby hospital and ask for a referral to a urologist. You can also call the local medical society and ask for a referral.

One thing you will want to find out about your doctor is if he or she is a board-certified urologist. In order to obtain board certification, a doctor must pass rigorous written and oral tests before peers in the field of specialization. In 1985, the American Board of Urology mandated that board-certified urologists be issued certification for a set period of ten years, after which time the urologist must go through a recertification. Recertification requires, among other things, submission of a statement containing any adverse actions involving licensure, hospital staff appointment, and malpractice litigation (past and pending), as well as the urologist's one hundred most recent operative cases or operative cases during one year (whichever is a shorter list) and other documentation.

Board certification is a *voluntary* program and a doctor

9

may have a good reason why he or she is not board-certified. Nevertheless, it is information that may be helpful in deciding on a urologist to see. Doctors who have board certification are listed in the *Directory of Medical Specialists*. You can usually find that reference book in the library. For a short cut, call 1-800-776-CERT. This is a service sponsored by the American Board of Medical Specialties. Someone will be able to tell you if your doctor is board-certified.

If cancer is suspected or you have been diagnosed with cancer, you may want to ask the urologist whether he or she specializes in cancer and/or how many cancer patients he or she generally treats.

THE VISIT

When you do go to see your doctor, if it is a first-time visit, he or she will take a complete medical history. You will be asked what illnesses you've had and when. You will be asked about cancer and other illnesses in your family. And you will be asked to describe, in as much detail as possible, the symptoms you are experiencing. It is a good idea to write down all you can about the symptoms, as well as questions, before you get to the doctor's office. It's easy to forget a symptom or two; and the more information you can give your doctor, the better.

You may want to keep a record of the symptoms that are occurring. It doesn't have to be elaborate. When you do keep a written record, you may discover that you are urinating much more frequently than you realized—or much less frequently than you thought. How many times do you wake up at night? Do you wake up about the same number of times each night? Even if you don't keep a formal hour-by-hour, day-by-day record, it's a good idea to write down all the different symptoms you're experiencing. It is easy to forget something that just occurred once or that you may think is not really significant. It is also helpful to be able to tell the doctor how long you've had the symptoms, whether they have gotten worse or improved, and whether they have been constant or episodic. Another bit of information that your doctor will probably want to know is how much liquid you generally drink each day, especially at night. The more information you can give your doctor, the more he or she has to work with.

It might be a good idea to bring someone with you—a family member or friend. This can help relieve some of the stress that frequently accompanies a visit to the doctor when a problem is suspected. It also gives you a second set of ears. The ideal person to bring is someone who is supportive, has a good memory, and is able to think objectively.

Bring a pad and take notes. You may even bring a tape recorder. Ask the doctor if he or she has any objections to your taping what is discussed. Explain that this will enable you to listen to what has been discussed and make sure you understand and follow the doctor's advice correctly. (This can also help family members understand what is going on when you talk to them later.) Even when you are not under stress, it can be difficult to understand and retain a lot of unfamiliar information. That difficulty is greatly increased when you are hearing things which may have a big impact on your life and the way you will be living in the future.

You may ask the doctor if there are any pictures you can look at to help you understand what is being said. If you don't understand something that is being said, say so! Some doctors are very good at talking in layman's terms that patients can understand. Others aren't. If you don't understand the doctor's answer to your question or think the doctor has not understood you, say so. And repeat the question.

QUESTIONS TO ASK

Following are questions you may want to ask your doctor. If you come up with some others, great! Not all of the questions will necessarily apply to your situation. They are meant to help you find out as much as you can about tests your doctor may suggest and the follow-up treatment, if necessary. For example, some routine tests can probably be performed by your regular doctor. There are other tests that require a specialist. There are diagnostic tests that are new and/or complex, requiring a great deal of expertise. You may not want to be the first or second patient on whom your doctor has performed such a procedure.

Before the visit, think about what you want to ask. It's a good idea to write your questions down. And ask them. If you feel uncomfortable asking the doctor *anything,* remember: It is *your* body and it is the only one you've got. The more knowledgeable you are, the better able you are to make the best decisions for yourself. (In addition, when you know what's going on, what to expect, you can deal with it. That knowledge can relieve a lot of anxiety and stress.)

Questions to Ask About Diagnostic Tests

1. Why is this test necessary?
2. What will it show?
3. How commonly is it performed? How frequently have you performed it?
4. How is it performed? How long does it take? Is hospitalization required? What preparations do I have to make beforehand? Does it involve any risk? What are the possible side effects? What is involved in terms of recovery from this test? How long should recovery take? At what point can I resume regular activities?
5. How much does it cost?

Questions to Ask About Treatment

1. What are my treatment options? Is there more than one treatment for this condition? If the answer is yes, what is the difference between them, which is better, which do you recommend, and why? What are the possible risks and side effects of each treatment option?

2. How commonly is this treatment performed? Do you perform it and, if so, how frequently have you performed it? What has your success rate been? If you don't perform this treatment, who does?

3. What is this treatment intended to accomplish? What can I expect in terms of results? (In the treatment of prostate cancer, the goal of the treatment may be cure, to shrink the tumor so that it can be treated by other means, reduce pain, prevent complications, or extend life.)

4. Is there anything I should do to prepare for this treatment? How is this treatment performed? How long does it take? Is hospitalization required? What preparations do I have to make beforehand? Does it involve any risk? What are the possible side effects? What can I do about them? What side effects should I call you about? What is involved in terms of recovery? How long should recovery take? At what point can I resume regular activities? What kind of follow-up will there be?

5. How much does it cost?

Questions to Ask if the Diagnosis Is Cancer

1. Are other tests necessary and, if so, why, and what are they? (See the earlier questions about tests.)

2. Has the cancer spread to any other place? If so, where has it spread to? What is the stage (extent) of the cancer? What is the cancer's grade (aggressiveness)?

3. What is the state-of-the-art treatment for my cancer? (See the earlier questions about treatment.)

4. Are clinical trials being done for my cancer? Do I qualify for any clinical trials and, if so, do you recommend it?

5. What is the prognosis? (This is your call. How much do you want to know? Bear in mind, there is *no* doctor who can tell anyone with certainty how long he or she is going to live. And statistics are just that—statistics!)

There are many, many kind, understanding, cooperative, and competent doctors. Some will routinely tell each patient all the relevant information. Some will not, for a number of reasons. What is important and relevant to you may be something your doctor may not see as relevant and so doesn't mention. Many doctors are very busy and if you don't ask, they don't tell. Some doctors aren't sure how much a patient wants to know and do not want to give information that the patient may not be ready to hear. It's up to you to decide how much and what you want to know and make it known to the doctor. Ask those questions. Again, many people feel it's helpful to bring someone along with them to the appointment.

Benign Conditions of the Prostate

Most benign (noncancerous) conditions of the prostate are just that—benign, harmless. But they can cause discomfort and pain. They can also provoke some high anxiety, as my friend Gus could tell you, and he is certainly not the exception. Gus is in his mid-fifties. A few years ago, he started having some discomfort in the groin area. He had to go to the bathroom more and more frequently. He always seemed to feel like he had to go to the bathroom, even if he didn't have to. "It wasn't painful or even an ache," he recalls. "It was more of a throbbing." Did he run to the doctor? Not right away. "I've always been healthy. I keep in good shape. I kept thinking it'll pass, it'll go away. I'm not one to run off to a doctor." Gus had not been going for a yearly exam, which he now says is "inexcusable." It had been years since he'd had a general checkup. Then he read an article stating that prostate cancer is a leading cause of death among men. According to the American Cancer Society, one in eleven men in the

United States will develop prostate cancer. The ACS estimated that approximately thirty-five thousand would die of prostate cancer in 1993. Gus panicked. A short time later he was in the office of a urologist, who performed a rectal exam as well as blood test and urinalysis. He told Gus to come back in two weeks. "Could it be cancer?" Gus asked. The doctor told him that it did not appear to be cancer, but added that the tests could indicate the possibility of cancer, in which case other tests would be performed. Gus was only slightly reassured. It was a long two weeks. In the meantime, the doctor prescribed the medication Hytrin, which is commonly used to treat high blood pressure and which is now one of the drugs used to treat an enlarged prostate. When Gus returned to the doctor, his symptoms were greatly reduced and he heard the good news. It was not cancer. He still takes a pill a night and today is feeling fine. The medication has caused no side effects. He sees his doctor every three months for follow-up. Gus's prostate story has a good ending—as many prostate stories do. But again, it is important to see the doctor whenever there is a problem and as soon as possible! And if you are forty or over, you should have a yearly DRE.

PROSTATITIS SYNDROMES

Prostatitis (the suffix *itis* indicates inflammation) is an inflammation of the prostate which may be caused by bacteria (bacterial prostatitis) or other conditions. It is a very common disorder and can occur at virtually any age, unlike other prostate problems, which usually affect primarily middle-aged and older men. Prostatitis can occur in a boy who is still a teen and in his grandfather! Although the symptoms can be very frightening when they occur the first time, prostatitis is generally not considered to be that serious and, depending on the type, responds well to treatment.

There are five conditions that come under the general heading of prostatitis. They are:

- Acute bacterial prostatitis (you may see this referred to as acute infectious prostatitis)
- Chronic bacterial prostatitis (you may see this referred to as chronic infectious prostatitis)
- Nonbacterial prostatitis (you may see this referred to as noninfectious prostatitis), which is always chronic
- Prostatosis
- Prostatodynia

Bacterial prostatitis is usually the result of an infection (caused by bacteria) that has spread from the urinary tract or another part of the body. Almost all men have bacteria in their prostate. However, few men will develop an infection causing symptoms that require treatment. Some men appear to have a biological predisposition that makes them more susceptible to the bacteria.

Bacteria can reach the prostate area in several ways—through the bloodstream, the lymph system, or the urethra. While it may be relatively easy for the bacteria to make its way to the prostate, it isn't that easy to get in. There is a blood barrier that keeps some out. (This same barrier can also prevent some curative antibiotics from getting in.) When the bacterial agents do get through, they can be successful in taking up more or less permanent residence. The prostate does not drain itself very well. The infection can dig in, making it difficult to cure. Bacterial prostatitis can be acute or chronic.

Acute bacterial prostatitis is the least common type of prostatitis. It comes on suddenly and its symptoms are severe. They include chills and moderate to high fever, back pain, and problems urinating. Immediate hospitalization is usually required. The most common cause of acute bacterial prostatitis is colon bacilli which can reach the prostate directly by way of the rectum or through the bloodstream. Gonorrhea can be a cause of acute prostatitis. Acute prostatitis is treated with antibiotics and can usually be cured.

Chronic bacterial prostatitis occurs more frequently than acute prostatitis, though it is also fairly rare. It can develop very slowly. It is not uncommon for it to develop after a man has had acute bacterial prostatitis. It can also develop when there is no history of acute prostatitis.

Chronic prostatitis can be caused in the same way as acute prostatitis—bacteria can reach the prostate by way of the rectum or through the bloodstream; gonorrhea can also be a cause. There are frequently no symptoms other than recurring cystitis, which is an infection of the bladder. Chronic bacterial prostatitis can cause extreme discomfort.

Nonbacterial prostatitis is about eight times more prevalent than bacterial prostatitis. It is the most commonly occurring form of prostatitis. As its name implies, it is not caused by bacteria. Although there are increased numbers of inflammatory cells present, no infectious agent can be found. Its cause has not been confirmed, and it can be difficult to treat. It is generally treated with antibiotics. However, successful treatment usually entails a treatment program tailored for the specific patient, to relieve symptoms as well as anxiety and concerns.

Prostatosis (the suffix *osis* indicates congestion) is a condition in which the prostate is congested. Like nonbacterial prostatitis, it is not caused by bacteria. (Some doctors use the two terms interchangeably.) In prostatosis there is more fluid produced in the prostate than is emptied by ejaculation. This can result in an enlarged prostate pressing on the urethra and preventing you from emptying your bladder completely. A cause may be irregular or infrequent emptying of the prostate gland. The prostate gland empties during ejaculation. If there is a reduction in the frequency of ejaculation, there can be a buildup of fluid. There is no "normal" frequency of ejaculation. The frequency of ejaculation needed to empty the prostate can vary from man to man. It can also vary in one man. There may be no change in a man's frequency of ejaculation but he may suddenly, for no apparent reason, develop prostatosis.

Prostatodynia, or pelviperineal pain, is the term for a painful prostate, although it is usually not the prostate that is causing the pain. It is seen mainly in men aged twenty through forty-five. There may be pain in the rectum or the perineum—the area between the scrotum and anus—which appears to be a result of a prostate problem. Prostatodynia may be caused by a muscle spasm in the pelvis, an inflammation in one or more of the pelvic bones, or may result from a disease in the pelvis. Often there are no findings in a physical exam or in laboratory tests. Many physicians think that prostatodynia may be the result of stress, anxiety, and depression. If you have prostatodynia, it is quite unlikely that any abnormality will be found in your prostate and you may be advised by your physician to seek psychiatric help.

RISK FACTORS

There are some factors that can put you at a greater risk of developing prostatitis. Those factors are if you:

- Recently had a medical instrument, such as a catheter (a soft lubricated tube used to drain urine from the bladder), inserted during a medical procedure
- Engaged in anal intercourse
- Have an abnormal urinary tract

There are some things you can do to reduce your risk of developing prostatitis and its symptoms. Some factors which may play a role in the recurrence of the symptoms of prostatitis include too much:

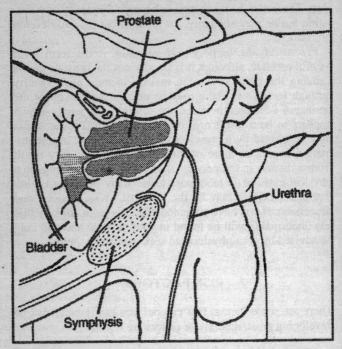

The prostate is symmetrically enlarged causing obstruction to urinary flow. (courtesy of *Primary Care & Cancer*)

- Coffee (of course, too much is different to different people, but one could safely assume your consumption is excessive if the coffeepot and your mug are always full!)
- Alcohol

While these drinks may not actually cause prostatitis, in some men they play a role in its symptoms, especially when the prostate is already in a weakened condition (very possibly from a previous bout of prostatitis). Very spicy food can also play havoc with a prostate that is not in the best of shape. And since having anal intercourse puts you at a risk of developing prostatitis through exposure to bacteria in the rectal area, either refrain from this activity or be sure a condom is being used. (Wearing a condom, or having "safe sex," is always a good idea because of the AIDS epidemic—which makes prostatitis look like a sniffle.)

The symptoms of the different types of prostatitis are often the same or overlap. They are also frequently the same as symptoms for other types of prostate disease, benign prostatic hypertrophy (BHP), and nonspecific urethritis (NSU). NSU is an infection in the penile urethra, the part of the urethra that is surrounded by the prostate gland. Symptoms may include some, all, or none of the following:

- Fever
- Chills
- Any difficulty urinating
- Difficulty in starting to urinate
- A sudden inability to urinate
- More and more frequent urination
- A sense of urgency so that it is hard to postpone urination
- Awakening frequently during the night to urinate
- Blood in the urine
- Burning or pain during urination
- Low back pain
- Joint or muscle pain
- Painful ejaculation
- Hematospermia—slight bleeding with ejaculation

- Pain or discomfort in the perineum, the area between the scrotum and anus

Because the treatment for each condition of the prostate may vary, it is important that a correct diagnosis be made.

DIAGNOSIS

Prostatitis (bacterial and nonbacterial), prostatosis, and prostatodynia have many of the same symptoms. Following are tests which may be employed in diagnosis.

Digital Rectal Exam (DRE)

The prostate of a man suffering from prostatitis may feel "soft" or "boggy," although that can be a result of other factors as well. In a patient with acute prostatitis the prostate will be tender and feel hard, irregular, and warm. While performing the DRE, your doctor will also check for any signs of cancer. (For more information on the DRE, see section on diagnosis of prostate cancer.)

Prostatic Stripping

Prostatic stripping (massaging) may be done by the doctor when he or she is performing the DRE or collecting urine for analysis. With his hand, the doctor massages (strips) the prostate gland, pressing gently but firmly on it. Downward pressure will force some prostatic fluid out of the gland and into the urethra. The fluid is then collected and microscopically examined for signs of inflammation and infection. This procedure is not especially painful but may cause some discomfort, depending on how sensitive your prostate is. (Prostatic stripping may also be done as a treatment for nonbacterial prostatitis.) Prostatic stripping would *not* be performed in

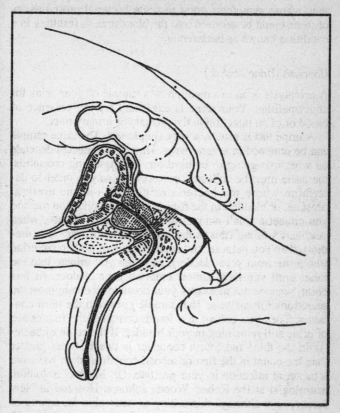

Examination of the prostate via a rectal exam. (courtesy of *Primary Care & Cancer*)

men whose symptoms point to acute bacterial prostatitis, as bacteria could be released into the bloodstream, resulting in a condition known as bacteremia.

Urinalysis (Urine Analysis)

A urinalysis is an examination of a sample of your urine for abnormalities. Your urine is examined for the presence of blood or of an infection in the prostate or urinary tract.

A urine test is usually a very simple test. The urine sample can be obtained in several ways. How it is collected depends on what it is going to be used for. In diagnosing prostatitis, the urine must be collected in a specific way in order to determine where the bacteria originated—in the urethra, prostate, or bladder. In the four-glass urine collection method you collect a small amount of urine, about an ounce, when you start voiding (this is the urine you void from your urethra), then you get a second small sample of midstream urine (the urine from your bladder), and then you urinate into the toilet until you have almost emptied your bladder. At this point, your doctor massages your prostate to obtain prostatic secretions for analysis. That sample goes into the third container. Then you collect in a fourth container the first ounce of urine still remaining in your bladder. If the count of bacteria in the third and fourth container is twenty times greater than the count in the first or second container, then you have a bacterial infection in your prostate. Dr. Michael Solomon, a urologist at the Robert Woods Johnson Hospital in New Jersey, says although this testing to determine the source of the urine is "useful in clarification of prostatic conditions [it is] often omitted in clinical practice . . . because obtaining the specimen is complicated, expensive and may not result in an important change in treatment." He adds that trying an antibiotic may be preferable to going through the complicated testing.

The presence of red blood cells in the urine can have a

number of different causes. It can be an indication of a mild inflammation in the urethra or bladder. This is not a significant problem. On the other hand, it may indicate a tumor, which has the ability to be life-threatening. Additional tests may be needed.

The presence of white blood cells (pus) is an indication of an inflammation in the urinary tract. In that case, a culture of the urine is done. A sample of the urine is put in a small dish which contains a nutrient on which bacteria, if present, will grow. The dish is incubated for twenty-four hours. The bacteria can be identified by its growth pattern. The number of bacteria present can actually be counted! In addition, different antibiotics can be put in one part of the dish to see which antibiotic is most effective against the bacteria.

Examination of all the samples will reveal whether your problem is an inflammation or infection and whether the problem is in the urethra, bladder, or prostate. Microscopic examination can show the presence of white blood cells, which may be an indication of infection, and/or the presence of red blood cells, which may be an indication of a mild inflammation—or cancer (a much more serious problem). If an infection is found or is suspected, a urine culture is needed for a definitive diagnosis. An identification of the bacteria causing the infection must also be made so that your doctor can prescribe the best drug for treatment. However, it is not unusual for bacteria in the prostate *not* to be found in the urine, so a negative urine culture does not rule out bacterial prostatitis.

Urine Flow Study

This measures the speed of the urine flow. It can help in evaluating the extent of urinary blockage. Additional tests such as an ultrascan of the bladder may be done to determine the amount of urine left in the bladder after urination.

If your problem is repeated infections (cystitis), your doctor may want to perform other tests, such as a cystoscopy or intravenous pyelogram. (For information on those tests, see the section on diagnosis/evaluation in prostate cancer.)

TREATMENT OF PROSTATITIS AND PROSTATODYNIA

Acute bacterial prostatitis is very responsive to antimicrobial drugs (antibiotics). Oral medications include ciprofloxacin, norfloxacin, and ofloxacin. Patients are generally on the medication for about two weeks. Patients with severe symptoms may have to be hospitalized.

Chronic bacterial prostatitis can be treated with antibiotics and controlled, but it is very difficult to cure. Sometimes the patient will appear to be better and will have been fine for several months when symptoms reappear. In some men it may be because they have what appears to be a biological predisposition that makes them more susceptible to the bacteria. These men lack what is known as the prostatic antibacterial factor in the prostate. The prostatic antibacterial factor is a zinc compound which appears to prevent the bacteria from becoming symptomatic. (Unfortunately, taking zinc supplements or injecting zinc has not proven to be effective as a preventive measure.) So when it looks like the prostatitis has been successfully treated, the symptoms can start up again.

Chronic prostatitis will probably need regular care. Patients whose prostatitis cannot be controlled or cured by medication may be candidates for a surgical procedure known as a transurethral resection of the prostate (TURP or TUR), in which the inner core of the prostate is removed by using an instrument inserted through the penis. TURP is only curative when all the infected tissue is removed. Because the bacteria often involve the capsule surrounding the prostate, which is not removed, only about a third of the patients who do undergo TURP are cured. (For more information on

TURP, see the treatment section in the chapter on BPH.) As bleak as this is, it does have an up side. Because the patient is seen regularly by his doctor, it is much more likely that if other prostate problems such as BPH or, more importantly, cancer develop, they will be detected in an early stage. This is especially significant in relation to cancer, as prostate cancer discovered very early in its development is frequently curable.

Nonbacterial prostatitis and prostatosis are generally not successfully treated with antibiotics because they are not caused by bacteria. Most men with acute symptoms will benefit from hot sitz baths. That is a simple enough treatment. You sit in a tub with enough hot water to cover the perineum (the area between the anus and scrotum). Soaking in warm to hot water to which various bath salts have been added can relieve pain or discomfort in the perineal area. Your doctor may also advise you to take an over-the-counter anti-inflammatory ibuprofen such as Advil, Nuprin, or Motrin.

Another "treatment" is increased orgasm and ejaculation in order to relieve the prostate of the accumulated fluid. This can be accomplished by sexual intercourse (believe it or not, there are people who really like this treatment!) or masturbation (there are people who like this treatment, as well).

Another way to reduce the fluid in the prostate gland is to go to your doctor for prostatic stripping. However, if this is a recurrent problem, going to the doctor on a regular basis for stripping, or massage, is not a very practical solution. It is time-consuming and costly. And there is little scientific basis for it.

Benign Prostatic Hypertrophy/Hyperplasia (BPH)

BPH is an enlargement of the prostate gland caused by an increased number of cells (hyperplasia) and/or an increase in the size of the existing cells (hypertrophy). (Most doctors use the terms interchangeably.) The condition is noncancerous.

The enlargement of the prostate is a very common condition and a natural part of the aging process. BPH generally does not occur in men under the age of forty-five. Fifteen years later it is very common. Over half the men in the United States over the age of sixty have an enlarged prostate. By the age of eighty, about eighty percent of men have BPH.

There is nothing you can do to prevent your prostate from enlarging. Many men with an enlarged prostate don't even know that it is bigger than normal until their doctor discovers it during a routine exam. And even then it is not a problem, because they are not affected by it. Or if they are, it is just a minor inconvenience, which is in no way life-threatening and which they can often live with without any treatment.

It is not definitively known why the prostate gland starts growing again when a man is over forty. It is thought that the growth is probably related to hormone changes during aging. One theory is that estrogen in the prostate gland may stimulate substances that promote the growth of cells. As a man ages, the level of active testosterone in his blood decreases, making the small amount of estrogen present in his body proportionally higher.

Another theory is that a substance derived from testosterone may help promote its growth. That substance is dihydrotestosterone (DHT). In most animals the ability to produce DHT declines as they age and they eventually are not able to produce it. Some research has indicated that with a drop in the level of testosterone in the blood, older men continue to produce high levels of DHT in the prostate. Men who do not produce DHT do not develop BPH.

And yet another theory is that cells are given instructions, or programmed by the body, early in life. Researchers say the cells in one section of the gland could "reawaken" later in life and deliver signals to other cells in the gland, instructing them to grow or making them more sensitive to hormones that influence growth.

Is BPH a problem? Not necessarily. It becomes a problem when it interferes with urinary functioning. How big a problem it is depends on the extent to which urinary functioning is obstructed. Urinary functioning is affected in about half of the men whose prostate gland is enlarged. One in ten men over the age of sixty has a serious urinary problem as a result of BPH.

When your prostate is enlarged, it can push against the urethra and bladder and impede the flow of urine. The result can be a variety of symptoms, virtually all related to the ability to urinate. In extreme (and rare) cases there is a complete inability to urinate. If this occurs, a doctor should be seen immediately.

A number of different factors enter into how serious a

problem BPH may become. The size of the enlarged prostate is generally less important than the *consistency* of the tissue. The prostate may be quite enlarged, but if the consistency of the tissue remains soft and flexible, you may have no problems. It's when the tissue gets tough and inflexible that a problem can occur.

Normally, the prostate gland relaxes to allow urine to pass through the urethra from the bladder. When the tissue in the prostate gland is not flexible, it is harder for the bladder to push the urine through. The enlarged prostate puts pressure on the urethra, squeezing it and narrowing the passageway. The bladder compensates by pushing harder, contracting more forcefully to get the urine through the urethra. The bladder muscle gradually becomes stronger, thicker, and more sensitive. This may be sufficient to keep the urethra open and allow the passage of urine. When it isn't, the flow of urine can be severely obstructed. And that is when it becomes more and more difficult to urinate.

Urinary functioning is what is most commonly affected by BPH. Generally symptoms will get progressively worse over time, although that is not always the case. You may have a sense that you haven't fully relieved your bladder. Your stream of urine may be weak. You may find it hard to start urinating, or that the flow is interrupted—it stops and starts. You may have to urinate more frequently than you had to in the past and/or find it difficult to put off urinating because the urge is so great. When you have that sudden sense of urgency to urinate at night, it is called nocturia. When you have nocturia, your sleep may be interrupted by the number of times you get up at night to go to the bathroom.

There may also be burning or pain during urination. That is usually caused by an infection in the bladder which can occur when the bladder is unable to empty all of the urine. The more difficult it is for the urine to pass through the urethra, the more likely it is that the bladder will not be able to empty entirely. When urine remains in the bladder, it stagnates and can become infected, resulting in a condition called cystitis. Cystitis, an inflammation of the bladder, is very common in women. When cystitis occurs in women it is generally harmless, although it can cause some discomfort. Cystitis occurs much less frequently in men—and can present more of a hazard. Because cystitis may be caused by a urinary tract problem such as an obstruction or tumor, the doctor will probably want to do additional tests.

A small percentage of men will develop acute urinary retention (a sudden inability to urinate) with virtually no advance warning. There may have been some partial obstruction without it bothering the man. Acute urinary retention may be triggered by taking over-the-counter cold or allergy medicines. Some of those medicines contain a decongestant drug known as a sympathomimetic. One rare but possible side effect is that it can prevent the bladder opening from relaxing and thereby prevent the release of urine. When there is partial obstruction, acute urinary retention can be brought on by alcohol, cold temperatures, or a long period of immobility. Acute urinary retention is rare and *very painful*. It requires immediate medical treatment.

More common is a gradual reduction in the flow of urine. The buildup of urine left behind in the bladder may become so great that the abdomen swells. (You may look pregnant!) When you cough, sneeze, strain, or laugh, some of that accumulated urine can dribble out. If this happens, treatment is essential. Without treatment, acute urinary retention may occur (very unpleasant), as well as bladder and/or kidney damage, bladder stones, and incontinence. These complications are relatively rare but are definitely something you want to avoid. See your doctor as soon as you have any symptoms!

Following is a list of the symptoms which may be an indication of BPH (or other disorders):

- A weak urinary stream
- A sense that your bladder has not been fully emptied

- Difficulty in starting to urinate
- Urinating more and more frequently
- An urgency so that it is hard to postpone urination
- Awakening frequently during the night to urinate
- While urinating, the stream stops and starts
- Burning or pain during urination
- A sudden inability to urinate
- A bloated abdomen with urine leakage
- Blood in the semen

Again, it is very important to see your doctor if you are experiencing any of these symptoms—so that you can nip any problem in the bud!

DIAGNOSIS/EVALUATION

Your doctor will perform various tests to diagnose your problem. Following is a brief explanation of the tests which may be performed.

Digital Rectal Exam (DRE)

The DRE is the first test that will be performed by your doctor. In BPH, the prostate tends to be symmetrically enlarged and feels rubbery to firm. There should be no hard nodules felt, which can be an indication of cancer. There should be no tenderness and no spontaneous urethral discharge, which can be a sign of prostatitis.

When you come in with symptoms typical of BPH, the doctor may not actually feel the enlargement. That may be because just the innermost part of the prostate is enlarged. The opposite can occur as well. During a routine exam, your doctor may find, to your surprise, that your prostate is enlarged even though you are experiencing no symptoms. (For information on how DRE is performed, see the section on diagnosis/evaluation in the chapter on prostate cancer.)

Urinalysis (Urine Analysis)

A urinalysis is an examination of a sample of your urine for abnormalities. Your urine is examined for the presence of blood in the urine or for the presence of an infection in the prostate or urinary tract. A urine test is usually a very simple test.

In testing for BPH, midstream urine is collected. Before urinating, you wash your penis with soap and water after pulling back the foreskin. (A man who is circumcised does not have to do the cleaning.) To get the sample, you urinate for a second or two and stop, then start again, this time collecting some of the urine in a sterile container. The flow of urine is then stopped before completion so that the container can be removed. Then the bladder can be completely emptied. This ensures getting as pure a sample of urine as possible for the most accurate evaluation—a sample that is not contaminated by cells or bacteria from the skin.

Urine Flow Study

This measures the speed of the urine flow. It can help in evaluating the extent of urinary blockage. You will be told to drink liquid in order to fill your bladder. The test is simply emptying your bladder into a special container that can measure and record the rate of your urine flow. If the flow rate is lower than normal, it is an indication that there may be an obstruction. In men under forty, the flow rate should be over twenty-two millimeters per second; between forty and sixty the flow rate should be over eighteen millimeters per second; and over sixty the flow rate should be over thirteen millimeters per second. Generally, the more below the normal flow rate, the greater the need for surgery. However, on occasion, the slow flow rate may be a result of a bladder problem and not an enlarged prostate.

Ultrasound (US)

This is a diagnostic procedure that bounces high-frequency sound waves off tissues and changes the echoes into pictures. Ultrasound can be used to find and measure solid tumors in the body. A bladder ultrasound may be performed to look for residual urine. (For information on ultrasound, see the section on diagnosis/evaluation in the chapter on prostate cancer.)

Blood Test

A blood test is the examination of a sample of blood. Blood tests are done in the detection, diagnosis, and monitoring of many different medical problems. In the diagnosis of BPH, a blood test will not specifically show BPH. What it can show is a high level of the substance creatinine, which can be an indirect result of an enlarged prostate. The presence of too much creatinine in the blood can indicate a problem with how the kidneys are functioning. Creatinine is a waste product produced by the normal breakdown of body muscle at a constant rate each day. It is the job of the kidneys to remove waste products, including creatinine, from the blood and excrete them in the urine. Too high a level of creatinine in the blood is usually the result of a malfunctioning kidney. The malfunctioning kidney may be a result of an enlarged prostate blocking the passage of urine and preventing the bladder from emptying fully. With treatment, normal functioning of the kidney is usually restored.

The amount of certain substances produced by the prostate can also be assessed in the blood. A higher than normal level of prostate-specific antigen (PSA), a protein which is made only by the prostate, can be caused by BPH or other prostate conditions. Some 30 percent of patients with BPH will have an elevated PSA. A very high PSA level can suggest the presence of cancer. An abnormally high level of the enzyme prostatic acid phosphatase (PAP), produced by the prostate and found in a blood test, can also suggest the presence of cancer.

Cystoscopy

A cystoscopy is a visual examination of the bladder and urethra in which a lighted, tubular instrument called a cystoscope is used. There are two types of cystoscopes. The traditional cystoscope is rigid. The flexible cystoscope is the newer, state-of-the-art model. The flexible cystoscope serves the same purpose as the rigid model but is less uncomfortable. As more doctors acquire the new, flexible cystoscope, flexible cystoscopy will be performed with increased frequency.

The cystoscope enables the doctor to actually see the extent to which the urethra is obstructed by an enlarged prostate, and determine the best surgical approach for removal of the tissue that is causing the obstruction. While performing the cystoscopy, the doctor can also check the bladder for any changes caused by the BPH or for the presence of any other abnormality or disease, such as an unrelated bladder cancer.

In performing the procedure, the cystoscope is coated with an anesthetic jelly and inserted through the urethra by way of the penis, which has also been lubricated with the jelly, and then into the bladder. Water is inserted into the bladder so that the doctor can get a better look at the bladder walls. Small forceps can be inserted through the cystoscope to pick up cells for biopsy (microscopic examination for cancer) if any suspicious area is seen. This procedure is generally done under a local anesthesia in the doctor's office. It can also be done under a general anesthesia in the hospital. It takes about fifteen minutes. And while it might not be the most pleasant procedure to go through, the numbing agent should prevent pain. At the most, there might be some discomfort. After the procedure there may be a swelling of the urethra, which could result in a temporary difficulty in urinating. There might be some slight bleeding (especially if a biopsy was performed) and there may be a burning feeling when urinating. These aftereffects could last a few days. You may be given a prescription for an antibiotic to take for a few days to prevent the possible onset of an infection.

Intravenous Pyelogram (IVP)

Also called an intravenous urogram (IVU), excretory urogram, or a KUB (kidneys, ureters, bladder), this procedure is an X ray of the urinary system using a contrast dye. It enables the doctor to see and evaluate the upper urinary tract (kidneys and ureters) and the lower urinary tract (bladder and urethra). An IVP can reveal problems which could affect surgery, such as kidney stones or blockage, before the surgery is performed. The bladder can be checked for stones which may have been caused by BPH. The IVP is also useful in evaluating the enlargement of the prostate. (For more information on the IVP, see the diagnosis/evaluation section of the chapter on prostate cancer.)

TREATMENT

Your doctor confirms it—your prostate is enlarged, you do have BPH. What do you do? Perhaps nothing. Treatment is only necessary if the symptoms are bothersome (what bothers you may not bother your neighbor!) or if the function of the urinary tract is greatly compromised. If you have symptoms that you can live with, you and your doctor may decide simply to wait and keep an eye on the condition. The doctor will check you at least once a year—maybe more often—for any significant changes and to make sure that you are not developing any complications from BPH. You may live that way without ever having the need for treatment. You may also recover. Studies show that in as many as one-third of mild cases of BPH, the symptoms clear up without any treatment.

If you do need treatment, there are a number of different procedures available. As of 1992, surgery was the most common treatment for BPH. Which surgical procedure is used is the one your doctor feels will be the most effective for you. Following are some of the surgical treatments.

Transurethral Resection of the Prostate (TURP or TUR)

TURP is the state-of-the-art treatment for BPH. About 90 percent of the men who are treated for BPH (about four hundred thousand a year) undergo a TURP. About 80 percent of patients respond favorably to this procedure. It is the second most common procedure paid for by Medicare. (Cataract lens replacement comes in first.) It is performed in the hospital and requires anesthesia but does not use an external incision.

A major advantage in the surgical treatment of BPH is that if you are one of the 80 percent to respond favorably, there is every likelihood that you will benefit right away. Your symptoms may be immediately alleviated. Or there may be a partial reduction of the symptoms, with a gradual improvement over time.

TURP is performed with an instrument called a resectoscope, which is very similar to a cystoscope. It is a narrow, lighted, tubular instrument about twelve inches long and half an inch in diameter. It has valves to control irrigating fluid and an electrical wire loop on the end that can cut tissue and seal blood vessels. The rectoscope is inserted through the penis and urethra into the prostate gland after the administration of anesthesia. The procedure can take an hour and a half.

During that time, fluid is being flushed through the recto-scope to keep the area free of blood and the obstructing tissue is cut away a piece at a time. The pieces are flushed out as the irrigating fluid is removed during and at the end of the operation. When the procedure is finished, a Foley catheter is inserted through the opening of the penis to drain urine from the bladder into a collection bag. The catheter has a balloon on the end, which is filled with water to keep it in place. The catheter usually remains for several days. Some doctors like

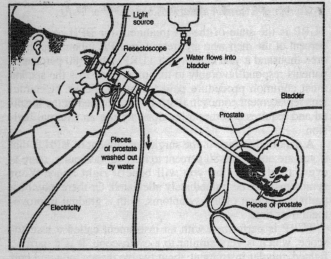

Doctor performing TURP with a resectoscope. (courtesy of *National Institute of Diabetes & Digestive & Kidney Disease NIH*)

it to stay in place for a longer period of time. The catheter can be irritating and may cause some painful spasms in the bladder.

You may be given antibiotics to prevent an infection. Or your doctor may want to wait to give you antibiotics, since not everyone undergoing a TURP develops an infection. TURP is a delicate and complex procedure requiring a physician who is skilled in performing it.

Your stay in the hospital can be anywhere from three to ten days. Your recovery, once you get home, can take about four weeks. A full recovery can take several months. You should discuss with your doctor what you can and cannot do. Although you may be able to have an erection, your doctor might suggest waiting until your internal incision has had more time to heal before you resume sexual activity. You should avoid any straining or sudden movements that could tear the incision—such as driving or operating heavy machinery, heavy lifting, or straining when you move your bowel. Drinking a lot of water is always a good thing to do, but it is especially important during this period. The water is necessary to flush the bladder. You may want to discuss with your doctor just how much you should drink.

The most common side effect, occurring in as many as 75 percent of the men treated with TURP, is retrograde ejaculation (dry orgasm). In retrograde ejaculation, some or all of your semen shoots back into your bladder during orgasm instead of exiting your body through your penis. The sperm is then eliminated from your bladder when you urinate. Retrograde ejaculation occurs because the opening of the bladder, which is supposed to slam shut during orgasm, frequently doesn't close completely after TURP surgery.

Retrograde ejaculation is not harmful, although if you are not prepared for this to happen—or even if you are prepared—it may come as a shock and be a bit disconcerting. It just takes getting used to. Retrograde ejaculation should in no way interfere with sexual desire or sexual intercourse. You have the same sensations during sex that you had in the past. The only difference is that you will not discharge semen through your penis. And for that reason, retrograde ejaculation will in all probability result in infertility, making it impossible for you to father a child. If this is a concern, you may want to discuss sperm banking with your physician before the surgery is performed. Sperm banking enables your sperm (male fertilizing cells) to be frozen and stored for future use. There is another possibility as well. Semen can be extracted from the urine if one voids right after ejaculation. In either case, it is then injected into the woman in the same procedure that is used in artificial insemination. (See the organizations appendix for more information on sperm banking.)

Other side effects of TURP may include incontinence, the inability to control urination. Although it is not that unusual to have some difficulty urinating for a period of time after the surgery, eventually you should be back to normal. A small number of men, at most 4 percent, permanently lose control of their urine.

Five to 10 percent of the men undergoing TURP may have difficulty getting an erection or be unable to get an erection after the surgery. The surgery rarely causes impotence. If you were suffering from impotency before the surgery, it would be extremely unusual for the surgery to correct that. On the other hand, if you had no trouble getting an erection shortly before the surgery, you should have no problem getting an erection after you've recovered from the surgery.

There are two other rare side effects that can occur. Scar tissue in the urethra or a narrowing of the urethra after surgery can interfere with urination. A narrowing of the bladder opening can potentially cause some urinary retention. So in rare cases, the curative surgery results in the same problem—but for different reasons.

TURP does not necessarily solve the BPH problem forever. There is about a 2 percent incidence a year of men who need to have the procedure performed again. When this happens, it is usually in men who were relatively young when they developed BPH, since it is usually about fifteen years from when the first TURP was performed when another is needed.

TURP offers some advantages over open prostatectomy, the other main surgery for BPH. Fewer days are spent in the hospital recuperating, and fewer days recovering. There is also less pain. A disadvantage may be that it requires additional skills to perform than are required for a prostatectomy. The size of the prostate usually determines the method used.

Transurethral Incision of the Prostate (TUIP)

This is a more limited surgical procedure that is similar to TURP and may be used in some cases. It is faster, simpler, and newer. It was first described by Ahmed Orandi in 1973 as an alternative to TURP. The same instrument used in performing TURP, a resectoscope, is used. Instead of removing tissue, the resectoscope makes cuts in the prostate and in the neck of the bladder where the urethra joins the bladder. The prostate gland splits to each side and relieves pressure on the urethra, restoring normal functioning. In most cases TUIP relieves symptoms of frequent or difficult urination fairly quickly. A plus: There is a much lower rate of retrograde ejaculation following this procedure. However, because this procedure is still so new, there are not much data on other side effects. There are also no data available on long-term efficacy and possible complications. For that reason, TUIP's role in the treatment of BPH is not firmly established. Because of its advantages over TURP, some doctors are convinced that TUIP will eventually replace TURP as the treatment of choice for prostate glands that are not greatly enlarged. Other doctors see only a limited advantage over TURP, since both require anesthesia. As with TURP, TUIP is not considered a treatment of choice for prostates that are greatly enlarged.

Open Prostatectomy

Open prostatectomy, removal of the prostate through an incision in the skin, is a more radical surgery. It has all but been replaced by TURP in the surgical treatment of BPH, with only 10 percent of patients having an open prostatectomy. However, the open prostatectomy is usually the treatment of choice when the prostate is very enlarged, because it would take too long to remove all the extra tissue when doing a TURP and absorption of the irrigating solutions used during the surgery limits the time allowed for performance of a TURP. An open prostatectomy may be the treatment of choice when there is also a problem with the bladder to be corrected, such as the removal of stones.

The prostatectomy is commonly referred to as an *open* prostatectomy because an external incision in the skin is required. In an open prostatectomy for BPH, only the gland is removed, with the capsule remaining in place. It is like removing the pulp from an orange and leaving the skin behind. It can be done in three different ways. Which way it is performed depends on a number of factors, including the location of the enlargement within the gland, the patient's size and body shape, and the preference of the surgeon. Following is a brief description of each method:

- *Suprapubic*. An incision is made through the lower abdomen and into the bladder. When the bladder is exposed, the physician puts a finger through the bladder neck and removes the entire prostate gland, leaving the capsule intact.
- *Retropubic*. The same incision is made in the abdomen so that the prostate gland is exposed and removed. This is very similar to the suprapubic prostatectomy. The major difference is that in the retropubic prostatectomy an incision is made in the prostatic capsule to remove the gland and not the bladder.

42

- *Perineal*. An incision is made in the area between the anus and scrotum and the gland is approached from below. This is the oldest and least performed method.

The recovery period for an open prostatectomy is substantially longer than for a TURP. It has the same side effects. As a result of the open prostatectomy the man is likely to be sterile. And there is a possibility of impotency.

The open prostatectomy differs significantly from a radical or total prostatectomy, in which the total prostate gland, its capsule, and the seminal vesicles are removed. A radical or total prostatectomy is one of the treatment options for prostate cancer.

Generally, surgery for BPH will solve the problem. However, when the bladder has already been weakened by the BPH, you may still have some symptoms—although they should be lessened. The thickening in the wall of the bladder does not always go away after the blockage is removed. The symptom that usually takes the longest to be eliminated is waking up at night.

There are other surgical treatments which are under investigation, including microwave hyperthermia (high body heat), laser surgery, balloon dilatation, and prostatic stents.

In microwave hyperthermia and laser surgery, tissue is destroyed instead of being removed and the end product is gradually eliminated by the body. Microwave and laser therapy appear to have the same result as TURP. A disadvantage is that because the tissue is destroyed, tissue cannot be examined for the possible presence of cancer cells. On the plus side, these investigational treatments can frequently be done on an outpatient basis. If the patient is hospitalized, he is usually released in twenty-four to forty-eight hours.

Microwave Hyperthermia

Two methods involving different ports of entry are being tried in the microwave procedure. The microwave probe can be inserted through the rectum or the urethra. The urethra route appears to be more effective than rectal insertion. A microwave probe called the prostatron has a cooling system. It keeps the urethra from being harmed by the high heat needed to destroy the surrounding prostate tissue.

Laser Surgery

In the past, the use of a laser to treat BPH was not considered useful. But more sophisticated laser equipment is now far more effective. In 1992 an Australian doctor reported that laser surgery using an Nd:Yag laser eliminated the urinary problems of all seventeen patients treated and that there was no bleeding in the procedure.

Balloon Dilatation or Urethroplasty

In this procedure a catheter is passed through the urethra to the prostate area. A balloon at the tip of the catheter is inflated to about an inch in the narrowed part of the urethra to obtain a wider opening. The balloon stays in this position for about ten to fifteen minutes. While this procedure does not require surgery, it is generally performed under a local anesthesia or spinal block. Although doctors are not exactly sure how this works, it appears that it may squeeze out extra fluid or it may break the capsule in which the prostate is encased, allowing the prostate to expand without restricting the flow of urine. Balloon urethroplasty requires a short hospital stay (usually just overnight), costs less than surgery, has a shorter recovery time, and has minimal side effects. It has been effective for four or five years in about 40 percent of patients treated with it. However, symptoms do return in many patients starting within a few months. Statistics covering a longer period of time are not available because this procedure has only been used since the late 1980s.

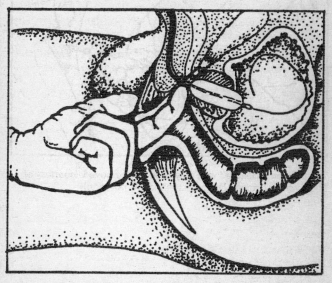

Inflation of the ballon in the urethra. (courtesy of Microvasive Urology Boston Scientific Corporation)

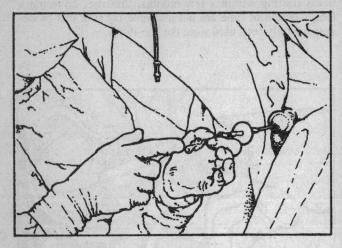

The balloon is deflated with a syringe and removed. (*courtesy of Microvasive Urology Boston Scientific Corporation*)

Prostatic Stent

Insertion of a stent—a thin metal tube—through the urethra and into the area narrowed by the enlargement of the prostate is being investigated in Europe. The stent expands and pushes back the prostatic tissue like a spring, thereby widening the urethra. The stent is a permanent implant. Eventually urethral lining grows over the stent. This procedure has had a good success rate. It may be particularly useful for men whose medical condition or age makes anesthesia and surgery a very high risk and are unable to undergo a TURP.

Efforts continue in order to find other, nonsurgical methods to treat BPH. And it does appear that those efforts may be paying off.

Alpha Blockers

Alpha blockers are drugs that do not reduce the size of the prostate but relax the muscle tissue in the bladder so that it is easier for urine to pass through the urethra. Alpha and beta refer to types of nerve receptors that maintain muscle tone. One of the alpha blockers being used in the treatment of BPH is terazosin (Hytrin). Hytrin is an antihypertensive medication originally used in the treatment of high blood pressure. It works by relaxing blood vessels so that blood passes through more easily, thereby lowering blood pressure. When Hytrin is used in the treatment of BPH, it relaxes the muscle tissue in the prostate and bladder neck, which can relieve some of the blockage, making it easier for the urine to pass through the urethra. It has a long half-life so that it only has to be taken once a day. Another alpha blocker is prazosin (Minipress).

The maximum dose that can be administered is generally the most effective. However, the higher the dose, the greater the side effects. Some of the side effects of alpha blockers may be dizziness or light-headedness, especially when getting up from a sitting or lying position.

Alpha blockers used in the treatment of BPH are still being investigated and are available only through a doctor's prescription. They have not yet been approved by the Food and Drug Administration (FDA) for treatment of BPH.

Proscar (finasteride) is a medication that was approved by the FDA in 1992. It shrinks the prostate by blocking the effect on the prostate of the major male hormone, testosterone. Proscar works by blocking an enzyme that converts testosterone to dihydrotestosterone (DHT), the active form within the prostate. It is DHT that stimulates the growth of the prostate. Because Proscar blocks DHT but does not eliminate or block testosterone, it is very rare for Proscar to cause impotency, as other hormonal treatments do.

In clinical trials, 50 percent of the patients treated with Proscar for BPH had a greater than 20 percent reduction in the size of their prostate and an improved urinary flow rate. It appears that the longer period of time one is on Proscar, the more the prostate's size is reduced and the greater the improvement in urination. Proscar is the only drug to date that will decrease the size of the prostate while maintaining potency.

Proscar was developed by Merck and Company over a fifteen-year period. Some physicians feel that if Proscar lives up to its potential, it could revolutionize the treatment of BPH. Merck predicts Proscar could eliminate the need for prostate surgery in some four hundred thousand men a year. Not everyone is quite that optimistic. Urologist Michael Solomon points out that it takes three months to see if the drug is working. In addition, there are some men who prefer surgery rather than having to take a pill every day for the rest of their lives.

Nafarelin Acetate

In a very small, initial study of the drug nafarelin acetate in nine patients with BPH, the enlargement of the prostate decreased in all of the men. During the treatment the men also had a reduced level of testosterone in their bodies. Nafarelin acetate is a hormone blocker that inhibits the production of testosterone by the testes by acting on the pituitary gland.

Prostate Cancer

CANCER: THE DISEASE

Before delving into prostate cancer, which is the most serious condition that can affect the prostate, a quick overview of cancer in general is provided.

Cancer is actually a general term for a group of diseases. There are over a hundred different types of cancer. Prostate cancer is just one type.

Cancer is a disease of the body's cells. Healthy cells that make up the body's tissues grow, divide, and replace themselves in an orderly way, keeping the body in good condition. When that system goes awry, the cells divide and multiply too rapidly without any order and a tumor develops. Tumors can be benign (noncancerous) or malignant (cancerous). There are several differences between a benign tumor and a cancerous tumor. A benign tumor does not spread to another part of the body. It can frequently be surgically removed and usually does not return. It is rarely life-threatening, although it can cause discomfort and harmful symptoms. (The major exception is a brain tumor. It is life-threatening because it has no place to expand in the skull and the pressure it exerts on the brain tissue can eventually result in death.) A malignant tumor can invade and destroy nearby tissue and organs. Cancer cells can metastasize (spread) to other parts of the body and start new tumors. If cancer is detected and treated early, before it has had a chance to spread, in most instances the chance for a full recovery, or cure, is very good.

The cause of most cancers is not fully understood. It is known that sunlight can cause skin cancer and that smoking can cause lung cancer as well as other cancers. It is believed that environmental factors, life-style, and heredity may all play a role in the development of cancer, probably in combination with each other to different degrees. For example, one may ask the question why some people who smoke a lot over a long period of time never develop cancer, while some people who have never smoked do get lung cancer. The people who do smoke and get cancer may have a genetic (heredity) predisposition which is, in some way, initiated by the carcinogens in tobacco. Or the smoker may live in a house containing the carcinogen radon (an environmental factor) or be exposed to radon in the workplace. People who smoke and are exposed to radon are at an exponentially greater risk of developing lung cancer than either the smoker who is not exposed to radon or the nonsmoker who is exposed to radon.

There are still many misconceptions about cancer. To many people the word *cancer* is simply terrifying. They equate a diagnosis of cancer with a death sentence. Jerry is not atypical. He was diagnosed with prostate cancer in 1985 when he was fifty-six. "My mouth just dropped. The word *cancer* hit me like a ton of bricks. When I heard the word *cancer*, I heard the word *death*." Jerry had been having some trouble urinating. When he saw a doctor, a TURP was performed for BPH. During the procedure, the cancer was discovered. When the doctor told him the bad news, his first thought was, "I'm going to die. I have to go home and talk to my wife and make plans." Jerry is now getting hormonal treatment, which he says is "giving me a lease on life."

Cancer is no longer an automatic death sentence. Today, half the people who get cancer survive. The numbers are even better for men diagnosed with prostate cancer. In prostate cancer survival rates have been improving steadily and have increased from 50 percent to 71 percent over the past thirty years. Diagnostic and treatment methods keep improving. Again, the earlier cancer is detected and treated, the better the chance for a cure. Prostate cancer is the perfect example. When it is found, diagnosed, and treated early in its development, it is virtually always cured.

Once cancer is diagnosed, it is then staged. *Staging* is simply finding out how extensive the cancer is. Is it just in the site where it started or has it metastasized (spread) to other areas of the body? For example, in prostate cancer, is the cancer confined to the prostate where it originated or has it penetrated the capsule in which it is encased? Is it in nearby lymph nodes? Has it spread to another organ?

Other information about the cancer is also sought after the diagnosis. How malignant, or aggressive, a cancer is it? What is the cell type? This is referred to as *grading*.

It is very important that cancer is staged, and as accurately as possible, because staging is the crucial factor in determining the best treatment. Other issues may enter into treatment decisions, but staging is the factor that carries the most weight. For example, in prostate cancer it is very likely that stage A prostate cancer will be treated differently from stage C.

The treatment of cancer is complex. Cancers in different locations in the body are treated in different ways. Prostate cancer is not treated in the same way as breast cancer. Sometimes just one treatment is effective in treating the cancer. When a malignant tumor is found and there is no other cancer present, its removal may cure the person of cancer. Other times a combination of treatments is used. After surgery is performed, there may be radiation therapy to destroy any remaining cancer cells, or chemotherapy (anticancer drugs) may be given for the same purpose.

Treatment may be done to cure the cancer, to control it, or as palliation to alleviate or reduce the symptoms. Whenever possible, treatment is done to cure the cancer. Treatment which is administered with the intention of curing the cancer may end up controlling it. Or when treatment is begun, its goal may be to control the disease. (Nobody gets upset if the treatment ends up curing the patient instead of just controlling the cancer, which does happen!) Eventually, when the prospects of a cure or control of the cancer are considered nil, palliative treatment may be given to provide relief from symptoms and improve quality of life.

There are four main types of cancer treatment—surgery (removal of the cancer), radiation therapy (the use of high energy to destroy cancer cells), medication (chemotherapy—anticancer drugs—and hormones), and biological therapy (also referred to as immunotherapy), the newest treatment for cancer, which uses the body's immune system to fight the disease. To get the best response, two or more different treatments are commonly used.

Surgery is the treatment of disease by removal of tissue, usually by some kind of cutting device. It is the oldest and still most common treatment for cancer, including prostate cancer. Until fairly recently, surgery was the only treatment that could cure patients with cancer.

Surgery is a localized, site-specific treatment which plays multiple roles in cancer. In the prevention of cancer, surgery may be performed when precancerous cells are found. The most common role of surgery in the diagnosis of cancer is obtaining tissue for a biopsy. In some cases exploratory surgery may be performed. In the treatment of cancer, surgery is used to remove the malignant tumor. It is not uncommon for there to be more than one surgical procedure for a particular cancer, and more than one way of performing a particular surgical procedure. Surgery may be performed palliatively, to alleviate pain, or to restore a bodily function. Finally, reconstructive surgery is performed to correct functional or cosmetic defects resulting from the original cancer surgery. A man who is unable to get an erection as a result of prostatic surgery (impotency caused by surgery is *much less common today*) may get a penile implant.

The most common way of performing surgery remains the use of a knife. A number of other techniques are now available, including:

- Laser surgery—the use of an extremely narrow, intense, controlled beam of light
- Cryosurgery—the use of liquid nitrogen or carbon dioxide to destroy a tumor by freezing it
- Electrosurgery—the use of a high-frequency current to cut tissue

Radiation therapy (which is also referred to as radiotherapy, X-ray therapy, irradiation therapy, electron beam therapy, or cobalt treatment), like surgery, is a localized, site-specific treatment. High-energy penetrating rays or subatomic particles are used to treat or control disease. Radiation therapy works by killing cancer cells and tumors, shrinking a tumor, or preventing cancer cells from dividing.

Radiation therapy dates back to the 1890s when the French physicist Antoine Henri Becquerel discovered uranium and Marie and Pierre Curie discovered radium, a substance even more radioactive than uranium. The development of radioactive cobalt, an artificial isotope that can deliver radiation therapy deep in the body with less skin irritation, made radiation therapy a much more viable therapy. Additional technological advances produced higher-energy machines capable of delivering radiation therapy even more deeply into the body with even less skin damage. As of the early 1990s, half the people diagnosed with cancer were treated with some form of radiation therapy.

Radiation therapy can be given in two ways: externally by a special machine or internally by placing radioactive substances in the body. Radiation therapy can treat cancer in most locations in the body. It can be used alone to cure some cancers. It may be used before surgery to shrink a tumor or after surgery to kill off any remaining cancer cells. It is also used frequently as palliative treatment to shrink tumors and reduce pressure, bleeding, pain, or other symptoms of cancer that cannot be cured. Radiation therapy is frequently used in the treatment of prostate cancer.

Chemotherapy is systemic treatment which travels throughout the body to find and eliminate any cancer cells which are present. Highly toxic anticancer drugs are used to cure or control the cancer. Chemotherapy destroys cancer cells by interfering with their growth or preventing their replication. Chemotherapy is used to a limited extent in the treatment of prostate cancer; its use in prostate cancer is mainly investigational.

Chemotherapy drugs must be approved for use by the Food and Drug Administration before they can be used on a regular basis for cancer treatment. Chemotherapy drugs are only approved after extensive testing in clinical trials.

Hormonal therapy is generally included under the heading of chemotherapy, although it treats the cancer in a different way. It is the use or manipulation of hormones and is a common treatment of prostate cancer.

Biological therapy, also called immunotherapy, is the newest cancer treatment. It is still primarily investigational. Its basis is using the body's immune system to fight and conquer the cancer. Substances occurring naturally in the body and others produced in a lab are used to boost, direct, or restore the normal defenses of the body. It is believed that biological therapy may be most effective when used in combination with other treatments.

CANCER OF THE PROSTATE

Prostate cancer is a condition in which cancer cells in the prostate form a tumor and invade and destroy tissue. The cancer can also affect surrounding organs and can metastasize (spread) to distant normal organs. When prostate cancer spreads, it most commonly goes to the lymph nodes and then affects the bones, especially the pelvis and lower spine. It can also affect other organs, including the bladder, rectum, lungs, liver, and brain. Over 95 percent of prostate cancers are adenocarcinomas, which means they probably developed in the glandular tissue located in the outer portion of the prostate. The remaining prostate cancers are very rare and include atypical adenocarcinomas, endometroid tumors, carcinosarcomas, and lymphomas.

Prostate cancer is the second most common cancer in men, after skin cancer. It is the second most common cause of death from cancer in men, after lung cancer. (In the United States in 1993 it was estimated that some 165,000 men would be diagnosed with prostate cancer and 35,000 men would die of prostate cancer; in the same year it was estimated that 100,000 men would be diagnosed with lung cancer and 93,000 would die). One in eleven men in the United States will be diagnosed with prostate cancer sometime during his lifetime.

Prostate cancer occurs most frequently in older men—the average age of diagnosis is seventy-three. Over 80 percent of all prostate cancers are diagnosed in men over the age of sixty-five. Only 2 percent of the cases of prostate cancer occur in men under fifty. Black American men have the highest incidence of prostate cancer in the world. It is not known why. Their survival rate is lower than the survival rate of white men with prostate cancer. There may very well be an explanation for the poor survival rate. It is believed that black American men have a lower survival rate, at least in part, as a result of later detection of the cancer and lack of adequate medical care and medical insurance coverage. Prostate cancer is more common in North America and northwestern Europe. It occurs much less frequently in the Near East, Africa, Central America, and South America. In Shanghai, China, there are 0.8 cases per 100,000 men; in Alameda County, California there are 100.2 cases per 100,000 men!

Although one in eleven men will be diagnosed with prostate cancer during his lifetime, many more men will actually have the disease but will not know about it while they are alive. At autopsy, some 50 percent of men eighty years old will be found to have prostate cancer. The incidence rises rapidly after the age of eighty. Only about 10 percent of those men will know about their cancer while they are alive. And only 3 percent of them will die of the disease. Most will die of unrelated causes with no significant symptoms of prostate cancer. Therefore, very few of the men who actually have prostate cancer will die of it. The older the man is when diagnosed, and therefore the shorter his life expectancy is, the greater the probability that he will not die from prostate cancer. This presents a dilemma as to how vigorously screening for prostate cancer should be, especially in older men, and how vigorously it should be treated, if at all, in older men. There are no easy answers. The course that any prostate cancer takes is influenced by a number of factors, including the stage and grade of the cancer when it is diagnosed, the age of the man, and the man's physical condition.

You are at a greater risk of developing prostate cancer if you:

- Are over 65.
- Are living in North America or northwestern Europe.
- Are black—black men have a higher incidence and higher mortality rate. But with an age adjustment, black men develop cancer about five years earlier than white men, and the incidence and mortality rates are about equal with those of white men.
- Have a first-degree relative (a brother or father) and sec-

ond-degree relative (an uncle or grandfather) who had prostate cancer.

In 1992, the National Cancer Institute's Division of Cancer Prevention and Control (DCPC) declared that DCPC will be placing a greater emphasis on prostate cancer. Bruce Chabner, director of the DCPC, told his advisory board that "while we frequently discussed the need for expanding our research base in breast cancer, prostate cancer has received one-fifth the funding of breast cancer, and at present we have few options other than hormonal therapy for metastatic disease." He said the DCPC would be placing a high priority on new initiatives in prostate cancer.

CAUSES

There is still a lot to be learned about what causes prostate cancer. It is believed that prostate cancer develops over a long period of time as a result of gradual changes in the cells. Although there is no single theory to explain the development of the disease, a number of causes have been suggested. Following is a brief explanation of each theory and its role thus far in the development of prostate cancer.

Genetic Predisposition (Heredity)

Data from population studies are inconclusive. Some studies have found what appears to be a genetic predisposition to prostate cancer, with an increased risk for blood relatives of men with the disease—and a three-times-greater mortality rate in the relatives of patients with prostate cancer compared with patients in a control group. Based on those studies, men with a first-degree relative (father or brother) and second-degree relative (uncle or grandfather) who have had the disease are estimated to be eight times more at risk of developing prostate cancer. In 1991 Dr. Patrick Walsh, urologist in chief at Johns

Hopkins Medical Institution in Baltimore reported findings in a study comparing the family history of 690 men with prostate cancer. His findings are outlined in the table that follows.

Relative Risk of Developing Prostate Cancer for Relatives

Number of Affected Relatives	Relative Risk
Father and/or brothers	
One	2-fold
Two	5-fold
Three or more	11-fold
Father/brother or grandfather/uncle	
One	1.5-fold
Two	2.3-fold
Three or more	3.6-fold

From *Prostate Cancer Update,* The Johns Hopkins Medical Institution, Volume 2, Number 1, Winter 1991.

Other studies have not shown such a familial link.

Until recently, there have been no chromosomal markers reported in prostate cancer. However, the tremendous advances in microbiology have resulted in new possibilities for understanding the basic mechanism of cancer. Prostate cancer appears to be, in many cases, associated with an abnormality in a genetic marker called P53 on chromosome 17. When this abnormality is present, regulation of the growth of prostate cells may be affected and the prostate cells may grow uncontrolled, like a car without brakes.

Hormonal Factors

Scientists have long suspected that hormones in some way contribute to the development of prostate cancer. It is unheard of for a man whose testicles were removed before puberty to get prostate cancer. The reason appears to be that the primary source of male hormones was removed. Researchers have induced prostate cancer in rats by the continued administration of hormones. Studies have suggested higher testosterone levels in men with prostate cancer than in those with BPH. However, the role that hormones play in the development of prostate cancer is still not clearly defined. In an effort to determine whether differences in the hormone processes contribute to the development of prostate cancer, one area of research is a comparison of testosterone production (male sex hormone) and metabolism in prostate cancer patients with that of their brothers and with that of men from families who do not have prostate cancer.

In 1992, researchers in California reported that an enzyme that acts on testosterone may play a role in the development of prostate cancer. Men in Japan, who have some of the lowest rates of prostate cancer, have less activity of the enzyme known as 5 alpha reductase than American men, in particular black American men, who have among the highest rates of prostate cancer.

Sexual Factors

The possible role of sexually transmitted viruses in the development of prostate cancer is being studied. There appears to be no link between sexually transmitted diseases and prostate cancer. Scientists are continuing to look for a possible viral connection. Some scientists have suggested that some viruses that cause genital warts associated with endometrial and cervical cancer in women may also be associated with the development of prostate cancer in some men.

Environmental Factors

Many studies have been done in the workplace trying to link environmental factors to the development of prostate cancer. Some studies have shown that workers exposed to cadmium, a metallic element used in welding, electroplating, and the production of alkaline batteries, may have an increased risk of developing prostate cancer. However, dietary exposure to cadmium—for example, from oysters—does not appear to put men at any greater risk. There is also some indication that rubber workers may be at an increased risk. Findings are inconclusive.

Life-style Factors

There are studies that suggest that a diet rich in fat may increase the risk of prostate cancer as well as other cancers. For example, there is a higher incidence of prostate cancer among Japanese men in Hawaii, who have more fat in their diet, than Japanese men in Japan. In Japan, an increase in consumption of milk, meat, and eggs has been accompanied by an increased rate of prostate cancer. In the United States, an analysis of prostate cancer rates from 1950 to 1969 showed that more cancer deaths occurred in areas with a high consumption of foods containing fats. A study done in Belgium using data from thirty-six different countries found a relationship between the per-person supply of fat from dairy products and lard and incidence of cancer of the breast, rectum, colon, lung, and prostate.

Benign Prostatic Hypertrophy (BPH)

Some investigators have suggested a relationship between BPH and prostate cancer. There are no definitive data either way. One large study indicated a greater risk for developing prostate cancer in men with BPH. Another study found no increased risk of developing prostate cancer in men with BPH.

PREVENTION

Since the cause of prostate cancer is not really known, there is little you can consciously do to prevent it, with one possible exception—your diet. There is evidence that as many as one-third of all cancer deaths may be related to the foods one eats. The biggest culprit: fat. The most beneficial part of your diet: fiber. By following some simple guidelines, you may decrease your risk of prostate cancer and many other cancers, as well as other disorders linked to diet, such as heart disease.

In 1990, the National Cancer Institute issued the following guidelines:

- Eat a variety of foods.
- Maintain a healthy weight.
- Choose a diet low in fat, especially saturated fat and cholesterol. Fat should provide no more than 30 percent of total calories of food consumed, and saturated fat no more than 10 percent. (Under the guidelines, the grams of fat consumed is a function of the total calories consumed and should be no more than 30 percent.)
- Use sugars in moderation.
- Use salt and sodium in moderation.
- If you drink alcoholic beverages, do so in moderation.
- Eat twenty to thirty grams of fiber a day, with an upper limit of thirty-five grams. Fiber can be found in the following foods: bread, pastas, and cereals made with whole-grain flours such as rye, wheat, corn, and oats; and fruits and vegetables, especially apples, peaches, pears, potatoes, peas, and beans.

The American Cancer Society (ACS) and the National Academy of Science have come out with similar guidelines. They recommend including foods rich in vitamins A, C, and E, such as dark green and yellow vegetables like carrots, tomatoes, spinach, apricots, peaches, and cantaloupes for vitamin A and carotene; leafy vegetables, whole grain cereals, nuts, and beans for vitamin E; and citrus fruits as well as other red, yellow, and orange fruits and vegetables for vitamin C. The ACS also recommends avoiding obesity and keeping moderation in the consumption of salt-cured, smoked, and nitrate-cured foods.

In the fall of 1993 The National Cancer Institute announced approval of a 10-year study using the drug Proscar in asymptomatic men to see if Proscar could prevent prostate cancer. The double-blind study (neither the physician nor the patient knows who is receiving Proscar and who is receiving the placebo) will enroll 18,000 men—randomized for either Proscar or a placebo. Proscar has been shown to reduce hormone levels but its role in controlling tumors has not been proven. Theoretically, Proscar might be expected to increase the risk of prostate cancer by increasing intraprostatic testosterone while reducing dihytestosterone. That is a concern of some urologists.

Proscar received approval from the Food and Drug Administration for treatment of BPH in 1992. (See the section on BPH treatment for more information on Proscar.)

SYMPTOMS

It is common for prostate cancer to produce no symptoms until the disease is no longer confined to the prostate gland. For that reason it is important to follow guidelines established by the National Cancer Institute and the American Cancer Society for early detection. They all recommend a yearly digital rectal exam starting at age 40 and an immediate exam for any man who has persistent symptoms. In 1992 The American Cancer Society amended its guidelines. It now recommends a yearly PSA test along with the DRE starting at age 50. Although neither a DRE nor PSA is conclusive, they can detect some prostate cancers which have produced no symptoms. If you are 40 or older you should go once a year for a digital rectal exam and go to see your doctor if you have any of the symptoms listed at right.

The following symptoms may be an indication of prostate cancer as well as other disorders, including BPH and prostatitis:

- A weak urinary stream
- A sense that your bladder has not been fully emptied
- Difficulty in starting to urinate
- Urinating more and more frequently
- An urgency so that it is hard to postpone urination
- Awakening frequently during the night to urinate
- While urinating, the stream stops and starts
- Burning or pain during urination
- A sudden inability to urinate
- Hematuria (blood in the urine)

Yes, these are most of the symptoms listed earlier for BPH, and indeed if you have these symptoms there is every likelihood that you have the benign condition BPH! So don't panic. But do check with your doctor.

A persistent pain in the back, hips, and/or pelvis along with fatigue and anemia may also be an indication of prostate cancer when there are none of the symptoms from the list just given. The pain is not a result of the cancer in the prostate but rather from the spread of the prostate cancer to the bones. When tests are done to diagnose the pain in your back, it may be found that cancer is causing the bone pain, but it is cancer that has spread from the prostate. If you are experiencing pain in the back, hips, or pelvis, see your doctor about it.

Because prostate cancer frequently has no symptoms when it is in an early stage and very small, it is not uncommon for it to be discovered by chance. For example, when a transurethral resection of the prostate (TURP) is performed in the treatment of BPH, some cancerous cells may be found in the tissue that is removed. Or, as just mentioned, some back pain may finally send you to the doctor, and the series of tests the doctor performs may discover that the back pain is being caused by prostate cancer that has spread to the bone. Your back pain may be the first symptom of the prostate cancer. However, back pain is a *very common* occurrence and can be caused by many different things besides cancer!

SCREENING/DETECTION

The ability to detect prostate cancer when it is in a very early stage is hampered greatly by the fact that symptoms are frequently not manifested until the cancer has already spread. That is why screening is important. *Screening* is checking for the existence of a particular disease in someone who has no symptoms. A mass screening will check a large population of nonsymptomatic people. Sometimes free screenings are offered. For example, screening for cancers of the prostate, skin, and breast may be offered at local health fairs, local hospitals, or by physicians who volunteer their services for a specific period of time. This is done to reach as many people as possible and to raise awareness of the value and importance of screening and early detection, since early detection of cancer offers the best chance of cure.

Screening guidelines generally target a specific population that shares common risk factors and will derive the greatest benefit from it. For example, checking a three-year-old child for skin cancer is pointless. It generally takes years for skin cancer to develop. In prostate cancer, the risk increases as a man ages. It is quite rare for prostate cancer to be found in someone under the age of forty. Therefore, screening for prostate cancer is generally directed at men aged forty and over.

The American Cancer Society, the National Cancer Institute, and the American Foundation for Urologic Disease all recommend that every man forty years of age and older have a yearly digital rectal exam. A DRE can detect abnormal conditions in the prostate which may be cancerous. It is presently the most accurate and cost-effective way to detect prostate cancer before it is symptomatic. Of the nodules discovered during DREs, 50 percent are malignant. It is estimated that some twelve thousand early *and curable* prostate cancers are detected each year by DRE. In 90 percent of the men whose prostate cancer starts in the periphery or outer part of the gland, a DRE can detect it.

If all men followed the guidelines, many lives could be saved. But it appears that many men are not following the guidelines. A survey by the Prostate Cancer Education Council found that nearly two-thirds of the 1,017 men questioned had not had a DRE during the previous year; more than 50 percent who did have a physical exam said a DRE was not part of the exam.

When a DRE detects an abnormal condition in the prostate that may be cancer, further tests are then needed. Two tests commonly performed are the transrectal ultrasound (TRUS) and a blood test for levels of prostate-specific antigen (PSA). A definitive diagnosis of prostate cancer can only be made after a biopsy is performed.

In recent years there has been considerable controversy over the role of TRUS and PSA levels as screening devices for the detection of prostate cancer. Some research suggests that transrectal ultrasound is twice as effective as DRE in detecting prostate cancer. It can detect small cancers in the prostate that cannot be palpated (felt) in a digital rectal exam. However, other doctors feel that though TRUS may help detect more cancers at an early stage, it may not increase overall survival rates and may simply subject many men to unnecessary treatment. They question its use as a screening device. As noted earlier, at autopsy, some 50 percent of men eighty years old will be found to have prostate cancer. The incidence rises rapidly after the age of eighty. Only about 10 percent of those men will know about their cancer while they are alive. And only 3 percent of these men will die of the disease. Most will die of unrelated causes with no significant symptoms of prostate cancer. In autopsies of men aged fifty who had never been diagnosed with prostate cancer, cancer cells were found in the prostate gland of 30 percent of the men. Therefore, very few of the men who actually have prostate cancer will die of it. It appears that though the ultrasound may detect the cancer while the man is still alive, he may very well derive no benefit from the very early detection of the cancer. In addition, the treatment he may receive as a result of the detection may do more harm than the cancer would have.

Ultrasound is a more time-consuming and costly procedure than the DRE. It requires special equipment and the ability to interpret the pictures produced. DRE requires no special equipment. Ultrasound can be a good complement to a positive DRE. It is also useful in locating palpable and nonpalpable tumors in the prostate for biopsy, directing the treatment of prostate cancer and measuring the size of the prostate.

An elevated PSA level can be an indication of cancer. In a study of some fifteen thousand men who underwent screening during Prostate Cancer Awareness Week in 1989, the PSA test made a very impressive showing. Of the 10 percent of the men who had elevated PSA levels, 40 percent turned out to have cancer; of the 17 percent of the men who had an abnormal DRE, 20 percent had cancer. In that screening, the PSA turned out to be about two times as effective as DRE. Other research has shown that up to 30 percent of prostate cancers that are localized (only in the prostate) have normal PSA levels. Elevated PSA levels can also be a result of noncancerous conditions such as benign prostatic hypertrophy (BPH), prostatitis, and other conditions. The PSA level can rise after any manipulation of the prostate, such as a DRE, biopsy, or TURP. Also, it is normal for a man's PSA level to rise as his prostate enlarges. These factors decrease the value of the PSA as a screening device. As with ultrasound, the benefit of finding prostate cancer at such an early stage is controversial.

If a PSA test is used for screening, it is most effective if it is done on a regular basis and the same test is used. A significant increase in the PSA level from one year to the next could strongly indicate the possibility of cancer. In the fall of 1992 The American Cancer Society recommended that men 50 years of age and older get a yearly PSA as well as a DRE.

The thinking has generally been that using the PSA as a screening device is not cost-effective. Its use in men who are at a greater risk of developing prostate cancer may be an exception. As with TRUS, a PSA test is very useful when performed after a suspicious DRE.

The PSA test is simple to do. A sample of blood is examined and analyzed for PSA. It is more costly than a DRE.

Although transrectal ultrasound and PSA may not be appropriate for general screening of prostate cancer, their use in conjunction with a suspicious DRE can be a valuable source of diagnostic information. (For more information on DRE, transrectal ultrasound, and PSA, see the next section on diagnosis and evaluation.)

A very new method of detecting early prostate cancer uses magnetic resonance imaging (MRI). A small probe is used in order to perform a transrectal MRI. This produces a high degree of resolution and sensitivity for prostate cancer as compared to BPH. Transrectal MRI could spare a patient an unnecessary biopsy. Its use in the early 1990s was not widespread; it is very expensive, far more costly than any of the other screening methods. With greater accessibility and a lowering of cost, the MRI may find a place in the detection of early prostate cancer.

There is some controversy in the issue of prostate screening. Most doctors do agree on the importance of screening for prostate cancer by an annual DRE. However, when you read further in the section on treatment you will find that there are times when treatment is not necessarily recommended after prostate cancer has been detected, for a number of reasons. Ironically, the screening goes up in importance as a man is younger. The younger a man is when early-stage prostate cancer is discovered, the more likely it is that the cancer will be life-threatening. It will have many years to grow and spread and eventually kill him if it is not detected and treated. The older a man is when he is diagnosed with early-stage prostate cancer, the more likely he is to die of something other than prostate cancer. Or he may die of prostate cancer but at an age when, according to statistics, he was likely to die anyway. Some, therefore, question the appropriateness of screening for *every* man forty years of age and older, as discovering the presence of prostate cancer in an eighty-year-old man may not extend his life.

DIAGNOSIS/EVALUATION

The purpose of performing tests is to get as much information as possible so that a correct diagnosis and prognosis can be made. Medicine is, at times, more of an art than a science. A test performed on one person may give clear and conclusive results; it is obviously positive or negative. The same test performed on another person with the same symptoms may give ambiguous information: the level falls in the "maybe" range; the X-ray pictures indicate the possible presence of some abnormality but could go either way. It is not that unusual for a test to be inconclusive, with results falling somewhere in a gray area. The test may be repeated or a different test may be performed to obtain additional information. Generally, several tests are performed in the diagnosis of prostate cancer. Occasionally a diagnosis can be made with just one test (that test would be a biopsy).

In cancer, a definitive diagnosis can only be obtained with a biopsy, microscopic examination of tissue or cells for cancer. And even then, the results can be iffy. Although it does not happen often in prostate cancer, it is possible that one pathologist (a doctor who specializes in the examination of normal and diseased cells) may diagnosis cancer, while another pathologist, looking at the same slides, may call the cells precancerous.

Generally, diagnosis and staging is done through a series

of tests. The number of tests it takes to diagnose an individual patient can cover a wide range. Sometimes two or three tests will provide all the information needed to definitively diagnose and stage the prostate cancer. Other times more tests will be needed. Which tests are used depend on the symptoms, the severity of the symptoms, the outcome of other tests, and other factors.

There are tests that may be done before a biopsy is performed to determine if it is needed. The tests may diagnose some condition other than cancer, so that a biopsy does not have to be done. If a biopsy is done and it is positive (cancer is present), other tests will be done to stage (evaluate) the extent of the cancer, to find out whether it is just in the place where it started or if it has spread into nearby tissue or into distant organs. In prostate cancer, the most common place for cancer to metastasize (spread) to is the bones.

The importance of correct administration of the test, up-to-date and properly maintained equipment, and correct interpretation cannot be stressed enough. (See the section on questions to ask about diagnostic tests in the chapter on you and your doctor.)

Diagnostic testing is also used to grade the cancer in order to get as much information on how the cancer might behave. This is especially important in prostate cancer, since autopsy studies show that so many men had cancer and never knew it. Researchers are trying to find a way to accurately determine whether the prostate cancer a man has will grow slowly and never cause problems or if it is the kind that will grow and spread rapidly and require aggressive treatment. Grading the tumor shows how aggressive the cancer cells are.

In grading, the cancer cells are microscopically examined to see how closely they resemble normal prostate cells. Well-differentiated cells most closely resemble normal cells, and poorly differentiated cells look very different from normal cells. Tumors consisting of well-differentiated cells are considered low-grade and have a better prognosis than poorly differentiated cells, which are considered high-grade. Grading refers to how aggressive the cancer appears to be and staging refers to the volume and location of the cancer cells in the body. You might think of grading as the speedometer in a car, telling how fast the tumor is growing, while the staging is the car's odometer, telling how far it has gone.

In addition to diagnosing and staging the cancer, some of the tests in the following discussion are also used to monitor how well you are doing on the treatment and as follow-up once you are no longer being treated. Many of the tests to be discussed are used in the diagnosis of other prostate problems and nonprostate-related conditions as well.

Following are the tests which may be performed in the diagnosis and staging of prostate cancer. It will be indicated when a test is more commonly performed in diagnosis, and when it is usually performed in evaluation. For example, a CAT scan and MRI are two tests that your doctor may want done if you did not have them during the diagnostic workup.

Digital Rectal Exam (DRE)

One could call the digital rectal exam the cornerstone of prostate cancer detection and diagnosis. The DRE is generally the first test used for any suspected problem with the prostate. It is a very simple, painless procedure that takes just a few minutes. Since the prostate is within your body, your doctor cannot look at it and examine it directly. However, it can be felt by the doctor during a digital rectal exam. This exam can be performed in several different positions. You can stand bent over, leaning your elbows on a firm surface, or you may lie on a table on your side with your knees drawn up. The doctor gently inserts a lubricated, rubber-gloved finger up the rectum to feel the prostate. DRE takes just a few minutes. There is no risk involved and no aftereffects. The doctor can examine the prostate for enlargement, lumps, or other areas of abnormal texture. The presence of nodules, firm, or irregular areas felt by your doctor may be an indication of cancer.

The DRE does not have to be done by a specialist. However, it is important that it be performed by someone who has had a lot of experience doing DREs. The accuracy of a DRE depends on a subjective evaluation by the examiner. It can be done by the doctor to whom you go for a yearly checkup as long as he or she performs it regularly. The more DREs a doctor has done, the more sensitive he or she is likely to be to any abnormalities. The American Cancer Society, the National Cancer Institute, and the American Urological Association all recommend that every man forty years of age and older have a yearly DRE.

If you feel uncomfortable and embarrassed about undergoing a digital rectal exam, you are not alone. Many men feel that way. Some will even avoid going to the doctor so that they don't have to go through the procedure, or will simply refuse to submit to it. I was surprised when one intelligent friend of mine in his early sixties told me with a pained expression that he'd never let any doctor do that to him. My advice to him and to you: Do it. Bottom line, it could save your life!

Blood Test

Blood tests are performed in the detection, diagnosis, and monitoring of many different medical problems. A blood test can measure things in the body such as sugar, cholesterol, antibodies, and harmful bacteria. It is a simple procedure, for you. A needle is inserted into a vein, usually in the arm, and some samples of blood are withdrawn. The blood is then examined and analyzed. There are several specific blood tests used in the detection, diagnosis, and monitoring of prostate cancer. Blood tests are objective tests that use automated techniques to measure results but require subjective interpretation.

Prostate-Specific Antigen (PSA) Test

The prostate-specific antigen is a protein produced by the prostate, specifically by the cells that line the surface of the ducts in the prostate from where most of the semen originates. It is known as a "tumor marker," because elevated levels can be an indication of a tumor. The PSA test is quick, simple, and generally painless. A small amount of blood is extracted, usually by a needle inserted into a vein. The blood is examined to determine how much PSA it contains. A very high level of PSA can be an indication of cancer. The higher the PSA level, the higher the possibility that its elevation is caused by cancer. However, an elevated level that is moderately elevated can be caused by many different conditions, including BPH and prostatitis. In fact, as a man ages and his prostate enlarges, so does the level of PSA in his blood. The PSA test is most useful when used:

- As a follow-up after a suspicious DRE. An elevated PSA will be further evidence of the possibility of cancer and generally an indication for the performance of a biopsy.
- As a monitor during treatment to see how effective the treatment is. A lower PSA level than was found previously is an indication that the treatment is working.
- As a monitor after treatment is concluded. An elevated PSA is an indication that the cancer may have recurred (returned).
- As a test of cancerous tissue at a site other than the prostate. The presence of PSA in the tissue can indicate that the primary site of the cancer is the prostate.

An elevated level of PSA in the blood during or after treatment is a red flag. It can indicate that the treatment is not working or that cancer has recurred.

The use of PSA demonstrates an interesting example of how progress is made in medicine. The PSA test was originally described in 1970 as a test in forensic medicine to document rape, since PSA is the enzyme that liquefies the semen and is made only by the prostate. Its presence in vaginal fluid could only come from semen. It was not until twenty years later that it was recognized that this same test could be used as a valuable tool for monitoring men with prostate cancer. Since the PSA is easily done once blood is drawn and is objective rather than subjective, the PSA has become the most useful marker for prostate cancer. In the fall of 1992 The American Cancer Society recommended that men fifty years of age and older get a yearly PSA as well as a DRE.

Prostatic Acid Phosphatase (PAP) Test

Prostatic acid phosphatase is another tumor marker which may be an indication of prostate cancer. This test was used since the 1950s and prior to the PSA test was the most useful blood test for prostate cancer. Prostatic acid phosphatase is an enzyme produced by the prostate and found in the blood. An elevated level may indicate cancer and/or the presence of metastatic disease. As with the PSA test, an elevated level can be caused by other conditions. And someone with a normal level can have prostate cancer. The PSA test is believed to be more reliable and more useful than the PAP test.

Ultrasound

Ultrasound, which may also be referred to as sonography or ultrasonography, is a relatively new way to locate and measure tumors in the body. It uses very high frequency sound waves which we cannot hear, just like radar. A small, hand-held device called a transducer (a device that receives energy from a system and retransmits it, often in a different form, to another system) is used to transmit the sound waves to a specific site in the body. The transducer is rubbed over the site to produce echoes. The echoes are transformed into pictures (sonograms) by a computer. Tumors, which give off different echoes than normal tissue, can be detected in the pictures. Ultrasound can show the presence of a tumor, its approximate size, and its local spread. However, it cannot show whether the tumor is benign or malignant. Ultrasound has several good features: It is painless, without risk, and can be done relatively quickly in a doctor's office. Ultrasound used in the diagnosis of prostate cancer can be performed in two different ways: transabdominal and transrectal, which is the most common method.

Transrectal Ultrasound (TRUS)

TRUS is the newer of the two techniques and is generally the method of choice. Although it's been around since 1971, its use was limited because it produced poor visualization of the prostate. With newer, high-frequency transducers, visualization of the prostate has been greatly improved. The size, shape, and general outline of the prostate can be seen.

The procedure is simple. You lie on your side with your upper leg rolled forward. The transducer is lubricated and inserted into your rectum. The transducer is slowly moved as the sonograms are made. It takes about fifteen minutes. This is neither harmful nor painful, although there may be some discomfort. The test is performed with the bladder partially filled.

The transrectal ultrasound has one big advantage over the transabdominal ultrasound. When the transducer is in the rectum, besides producing the sound waves, it can guide needles for the removal of some tissue from the prostate for a biopsy (microscopic examination of cells for cancer). This can be done without anesthesia.

TRUS allows for more accurate staging because the cancer can be measured more precisely. However, it cannot assess a stage D prostate cancer because it doesn't visualize regional lymph nodes. And it cannot distinguish between stages C and B because it is unable to show, with accuracy, involvement of the capsule containing the prostate.

Transrectal ultrasound is also being used by some doctors to screen for prostate cancer in men without symptoms. Its use as a screening device is controversial. Transrectal ultrasound is more time-consuming, complicated, and costly than a digital rectal exam.

Transabdominal Ultrasound

This method is the older of the two methods. Before the procedure begins, you must drink four or five glasses of liquid in order to extend your abdomen. When you are ready for the procedure, you lie on a table and a lubricant is put on your stomach. The transducer is then rubbed back and forth over the area where the prostate is located and the sonograms are taken. This takes about half an hour and is not painful, although there may be some discomfort from all that liquid you drank. The transabdominal ultrasound can also be used to assess the kidneys in men with bladder outlet obstruction.

Biopsy

A biopsy is the microscopic examination of fluid, tissue, or cells removed from the body to determine if cancer cells are present. A pathologist (a doctor who specializes in the diagnosis of disease by studying cells and tissues removed from the body) examines the tissue under a microscope to see if there are any cancer cells, and if there are, what type. Generally a biopsy is the only way to get a definitive diagnosis of cancer. The two biopsies most commonly performed in the diagnosis of prostate cancer are the core-needle biopsy and the transrectal fine-needle aspiration biopsy. During these procedures a transrectal ultrasound may be used to guide the needle.

If the biopsy is positive (cancer is present) the tissue may also be used to grade the cancer cells, and flow cytometry may be performed.

Core-Needle Biopsy

This procedure is also known as a needle biopsy, a wide-core needle biopsy, and punch biopsy. A special needle which contains a minuscule cutting instrument is used. In a core-needle biopsy of the prostate the needle may be inserted by one of two routes: through the area between the scrotum and anus (a transperineal biopsy) or through the rectum (transrectal biopsy).

The transrectal is preferred because a smaller needle is used and your skin is not penetrated. Once the needle is inserted, a small sample of tissue is removed. It takes about fifteen minutes and is not particularly painful. There are no lasting or major side effects. It can often be performed in the urologist's office.

The transperineal biopsy is a more difficult and painful procedure. Usually a general anesthetic is used and it is performed in a hospital setting, if only for the day. When the needle is inserted, a small sample of tissue is taken from the prostate. It takes about fifteen minutes, but you'll probably feel discomfort, maybe even some pain, for several days after the procedure.

Transrectal Fine-Needle Aspiration Biopsy

This procedure is also known as a needle biopsy, fine-needle aspiration MRI, magnetic resonance imaging, (FNA), and fine-needle biopsy. It is performed with a special needle which is smaller than the needle used in a core-needle biopsy. The needle is inserted through the rectum and into the prostate, from which a small tissue sample is removed. It has several advantages. It is usually done in the urologist's office and generally does not require anesthesia. Multiple samples of tissue can be obtained from different locations in the prostate. Fine-needle aspiration is being used more and more as physicians are trained in the technique and acquire skill in its execution, and as pathologists develop expertise in its interpretation. It is a relatively simple procedure which causes minimal discomfort and has a high level of accuracy.

Biopty Gun Biopsy

This is the newest, high-tech method of performing a prostate biopsy. It uses an intermediate-caliber needle which is thinner than the needle used for a traditional core-needle biopsy. The tissue is obtained with a spring-loaded biopty "gun." This technique also has several advantages. Precise samples of tissue can be obtained quickly with little discomfort. With the thinner needle, there is easier access for either a transrectal or transperineal biopsy and less bleeding. Anesthesia is not used. If the area in the prostate to be biopsied can be felt, the biopty gun is used alongside the finger. If the suspicious area cannot be felt, the biopty gun is inserted into a transrectal ultrasound probe. In addition, multiple tissue samples can be obtained, increasing the likelihood that if cancer is present, it will be detected. The biopty gun method seems to be replacing both the core-needle biopsy and fine-needle aspiration biopsy.

Flow Cytometry

This procedure, which is relatively new, is another way of assessing the cancer cells. It measures the amount of DNA (genetic material) in the cells. The DNA content is called ploidy. A tumor cell can have a normal amount of DNA (DNA diploid) or an abnormal amount of DNA (DNA aneuploid), too much or too little. Flow cytometry is performed on cancer cells that have been removed from the body. A fluorescent dye that attaches to DNA is added to the cells. A flow cytometer (a sophisticated laser-powered instrument with a computer system and terminal) then measures the amount of DNA on the cells. It is possible to identify characteristics of cancer cells that appear to be related to aggressiveness of the cancer (growth rate and potential to spread). The presence of aneuploid cells may indicate a more aggressive cancer with a greater risk of a recurrence (return) of prostate cancer.

Bone Scan

A bone scan is a nuclear imaging procedure which uses a radioactive tracer substance which is injected into the body. Once prostate cancer has been diagnosed, a bone scan can help determine if it has spread to the bones, a place to which prostate cancer frequently metastasizes (spreads). Areas in the bone with cancer will pick up more of the substance. It will appear as "hot spots" on the film. Those hot spots may be an indication of cancer. However, other conditions such as arthritis, infection, or a prior bone injury can also show up as hot spots.

A bone scan can look at the entire skeleton or one part of the body. If the bone scan is to examine a specific part of the body, the appropriate substance that will go to that site is injected. Once the radioactive tracer substance is injected, there can be a wait of two to four hours before the scan begins so that the substance can get to where it's going. During the scan you are lying on a table and—again—not moving. If the entire skeleton is done, which is usually the case, it can take about an hour.

This test is not painful and the only discomfort is not being able to move. It can be pretty boring. Sometimes you can see the pictures that are being taken on a monitor above you, which can make it a bit more interesting.

A bone scan is generally done after the diagnosis of prostate cancer to see if the cancer has spread to the bones. However, sometimes a bone scan that is taken to find out the cause of pain in an area of the body will show cancer that has metastasized from the prostate—before it is known that the man has prostate cancer.

Open Pelvic Lymph Node Dissection (Pelvic Lymphadenectomy)

In this procedure, used in the staging of prostate cancer, the lymph nodes are surgically removed and then biopsied. (Lymph nodes are small, bean-shaped structures that are found throughout the body; they produce and store infection-

and cancer-fighting cells.) This can be done at the same time as a radical prostatectomy or before the radical prostatectomy is performed. This can show a metastasis (spread) of cancer to the nearby lymph nodes in patients who are thought to have cancer that is confined to the prostate. This can be a strong determinant in whether aggressive surgical or radiation treatment for a cure should be performed. A diagnosis of positive lymph nodes will frequently eliminate aggressive surgery—which would not be a cure if the cancer has spread to the lymph nodes. It is the most accurate procedure for detecting lymph node involvement. It is also the most invasive and riskiest procedure for detecting nodal involvement. Pelvic lymph node dissection is a major surgical procedure. Because it contains some risk, doctors are not in full agreement about how appropriate it is for all patients diagnosed with prostate cancer. A biopsy of tissue in the lymph nodes is the only definitive way to determine if the cancer has metastasized to the lymph nodes. However, if a bone scan shows that the cancer has already spread to the bone, a lymph node assessment is not necessary. Whether the cancer has spread to the lymph nodes or other organs is a major determinant of subsequent treatment. (See also retropubic prostatectomy in the treatment section under "surgery" in this chapter.)

Laparoscopic Pelvic Lymph Node Dissection (LPLND; Laparoscopic Lymphadenectomy)

This is a nonsurgical procedure used to examine the lymph nodes in the staging of prostate cancer. It is a relatively new way of performing the more invasive open pelvic lymph node dissection just described. A laparoscope (a lighted tubular instrument in which forceps can be inserted) is passed through a small incision. The forceps are used to remove lymph nodes for biopsy. The LPLND is less invasive (the incisions made for the laparoscope are very small) and less painful than open pelvic lymph node dissection. It also carries less risk than the open pelvic lymph node dissection.

However, it has some disadvantages. It is a technique that requires additional training for the surgeon. Until the surgeon gains expertise in the procedure, it can take four to five hours to complete, requiring a long time under anesthesia. A study reported in 1992 which compared both methods in a relatively small sample of men found similar results for both. This procedure is not yet widely available.

Chest X Ray

An X ray of the chest can indicate whether prostate cancer has spread to the lungs, usually a late development after the cancer has spread to the lymph nodes and bone.

Intravenous Pyelogram (IVP)

An IVP is also known as an intravenous urography (IVU), excretory urogram, and pyelogram. It is an X-ray examination of the urinary system, kidneys, ureters, and bladder with the aid of a contrast media. A contrast media, also called a contrast dye, is a substance that will temporarily allow X-ray visualization of an organ so that X-ray pictures can be better interpreted. Before you're given the contrast media, an X ray is taken of your abdomen while you lie on your back. Then the contrast substance is injected into a vein in your arm. You may briefly feel flushed or nauseous. The dye travels through the body and outlines the kidneys, bladder, and ureters, and additional pictures are taken at ten- and twenty-minute intervals. A final X ray will be taken after you empty your bladder. The whole procedure usually takes an hour or less. There may be some discomfort but no pain. This can be done in a doctor's office.

An IVP can reveal obstructions or abnormalities in the kidneys, bladder, or ureters and help the doctor determine whether your symptoms are caused by a problem in the prostate or in the urinary tract.

IVPs were originally called Swick tests. Dr. Moses

Swick introduced the use of contrast dye in the United States in 1929.

CAT (Computerized Axial Tomography) Scan and CT (Computed Tomography) Scan

A CAT scan is commonly referred to as a CT scan and is also known as a computerized transaxial tomography and computed tomography. It is a relatively new procedure. It was first used in 1972. You could say that a CAT scan is an upgraded or high-tech X ray. The pictures are about a hundred times more sensitive. A CAT scan uses a computer to process the X rays. Highly detailed cross-sectional images (slices) of specific parts of the body, such as the pelvis, are produced. The pictures have a 3-D quality and show very small differences that are present in tissue. The CAT scan is not useful in the detection of prostate cancer. It may be performed in the staging of the cancer if lymph node involvement is suspected. The CAT scan can show enlarged lymph nodes. However, while enlarged lymph nodes are an indication of cancer, there can be other reasons for their enlargement.

Most of the time when a CAT scan of the pelvis is done (in order to see the prostate), a contrast dye is used. The dye is injected into a vein and then travels to the urine in your bladder. The dye enables even more detailed pictures to be taken, so that more information is obtained. During the CAT scan you lie on your back on a table. You don't move, but the table you're on does. It goes through what looks like a huge donut. The pictures are taken when the part of your body to be examined is located within the donut. As with a conventional X ray, you are told to hold your breath when the picture is being taken. After each picture is taken, the table will move a quarter or half inch so that a different slice of the area can be taken.

The scan itself takes about ten minutes and is in no way painful (except, possibly, the injection). A CAT scan can be done in the doctor's office. It may be administered by a trained technician, but the films, or pictures, are read by a radiologist.

Magnetic Resonance Imaging (MRI)

MRI is the very latest in high-tech imaging, and the most expensive. MRI was originally called nuclear magnetic resonance. In 1946 two Americans demonstrated its basic principle. They used MRI to analyze small chemical samples by exposing them to magnetic fields. In the mid-1970s a British company produced the first MRI of a human head. In the early 1980s it was rare to hear the letters MRI, even in medical circles, and it was difficult to find a hospital or radiologist who had the equipment. In 1989 there were twelve hundred MRI scanners operating in the United States. Today it is rare to find someone who hasn't heard of an MRI, although not everyone is completely sure just what it is and does. And today it is fairly rare to find a facility that does not have the equipment to perform an MRI.

MRI produces internal pictures of the body using powerful electromagnets, radio frequency waves, and a computer. It uses no radiation. It can produce highly resolute images of blood vessels, blood flow, cerebrospinal fluid, cartilage, bone marrow, muscles, ligaments, and the spinal cord. When an MRI of the prostate is done, it can show enlargement of the lymph glands, but it cannot identify microscopic spread of the cancer. An MRI can be done with a contrast dye, but that usually isn't necessary.

Because of those powerful electromagnets, you cannot have an MRI if you have a pacemaker, joint pins, surgical metal clips, artificial heart valves, shrapnel, or any other electronic or metal implant. As with other imaging procedures, you lie on a table—again, no moving—and let the MRI do the work. The MRI equipment, like the CAT scanner, is shaped like a huge donut. Like the CAT scan procedure, the table is wheeled through the donut to the point where the part of your body to be examined is within the donut. When you are wheeled into it, it is like going into a tunnel. Some people feel claustrophobic. It is also noisy, very noisy, when the pictures are being made, although as new, improved machines are being manufactured the noise level is decreasing. Each time a picture is taken, you hear clanging. It sounds like a jackhammer. Ask for earplugs. Some facilities have headphones so you can listen to music.

An MRI can take anywhere from half an hour to an hour. It is not painful, but it may be uncomfortable lying still for that length of time.

The MRI is generally not used in the diagnosis of prostate cancer. It may be used in the staging of prostate cancer. It can complement other tests and/or provide new and valuable information.

A very new use for the MRI is in the early detection of prostate cancer. Small probes have been developed which can be used for a transrectal MRI. A high degree of resolution and sensitivity for prostate cancer has been shown. This could prevent unnecessary biopsies. Its use in this capacity was not widespread in the early 1990s. However, with greater accessibility and a lowering of the cost (MRIs are very expensive), it may be used increasingly in the detection of early prostate cancer.

Transrectal MRI is also useful in staging. It is the most sensitive test, other than surgery, to determine spread of the disease through the prostatic capsule or into seminal vesicles, factors that would affect choice of treatment.

STAGES

Once prostate cancer is diagnosed, it is staged using the information provided by the tests that were administered. The stage of any cancer tells how extensive the cancer is.

There are several staging systems available. The most commonly used system in the United States is the American

Urologic System, which has been available since 1956. Another is the TNM (tumor-nodes-metastases) system. These are used with the Gleason grading system.

The American Urologic System uses the letters A, B, C, and D for the different stages. It then breaks down each stage into a substage based on the extent of disease and/or the degree of differentiation. *Differentiation* is a term used to describe or grade the cells in the malignant tumor. The more differentiated the cells are, the more like normal cells they are, and the *less* aggressive (fast growing) they are. Poorly differentiated cells are disorganized and abnormal-looking. They grow faster than well-differentiated cells. Following are the stages of the American Urologic System:

Stage A—Microscopic clusters of cancer cells are discovered incidentally in tissue samples removed during the surgical treatment for benign disease (BPH), a prostate cancer which *cannot* be detected by the doctor during a digital rectal exam.

> *Stage A1*—The tumor cells are well differentiated and are found in only one area of the prostate.
>
> *Stage A2*—The tumor cells are poorly differentiated or they occur in many areas of the prostate.

Stage B—The cancer is confined within the capsule of the prostate; it can be felt by the doctor during a digital rectal exam.

> *Stage B1*—A tumor that is no greater than 1.5 centimeters (less than five-eighths of an inch) in size is found in one lobe of the prostate.
>
> *Stage B2*—The cancer is more extensive, involving one or both lobes of the prostate.

Stage C—The cancer extends through the prostate capsule to nearby tissue, such as the seminal vesicles (the glands that produce semen), back of the bladder, or rectum.

> *Stage C1*—There is minimal extension to tissues surrounding the prostate.

Stage C2—There is more extensive spread to nearby tissues, often causing urinary obstruction.

Stage D—The cancer has spread to regional lymph nodes or beyond the pelvis to the bone or other organs.

Stage D0—The patient has no clinical symptoms of metastasis (spread of disease) but has a persistently elevated PAP level.

Stage D1—The cancer has spread only to distant lymph nodes.

Stage D2—The cancer has spread to distant lymph nodes, the bone, or other distant organs.

Stage D3—The cancer has progressed after hormonal therapy for advanced disease.

The tumor-nodes-metastases (TNM) system was devised by the American Joint Committee on Cancer. The *T* stands for tumor, the *N* stands for lymph node involvement, and the *M* stands for metastases. A number following the letter indicates the size of the tumor, the extent of lymph node involvement, and the extent of metastatic disease. The TNM stages correspond roughly to the letter stages on the American Urologic System. The corresponding letter from that system is in parentheses after the TNM stage. Following are the TNM stages of prostate cancer:

Stage T1 (A)—The tumor cannot be felt by the doctor during a digital rectal exam.

Stage T-1a (A)—No more than three areas of microscopic tumor cells are found.

Stage T-1b (A)—There are more than three areas of microscopic tissue found.

Stage T-2 (B)—The tumor can be palpated (felt).

Stage T-2a (B1)—The tumor is 1.5 centimeters or less and is surrounded by normal tissue.

Stage T-2b (B2)—The tumor is bigger than 1.5 centimeters or is in more than one lobe.

Stage T-3 (C)—The cancer extends into or beyond the capsule of the prostate.

Stage T-3a (C)—The tumor extends into the tissue surrounding the prostate or is in one seminal vessel.

Stage T-3b (C)—The tumor extends into the tissue surrounding the prostate and involves one or both seminal vesicles; tumor is more than six centimeters in size.

Stage T-4 (C)—The tumor is fixed or invades neighboring structures.

Stage N-1 (D1)—The tumor has spread to one lymph node and is no larger than two centimeters in size.

Stage N-2 (D1)—The tumor has spread to a single lymph node and is more than two centimeters but less than five centimeters in size, or has spread to multiple lymph nodes, none more than five centimeters in size.

Stage N-3 (D2)—The tumor has spread to one or more lymph nodes and is larger than five centimeters in size.

Stage M-1 (D2)—The tumor has spread to distant sites.

The Gleason grading system is a way of describing prostate cancer based on the appearance of the cancer cells and their degree of differentiation. The more differentiated, the more the cell is like a normal prostate cell and the less aggressive (fast growing) it is. The Gleason scale is the best-known grading system for prostate cancer. Following is how the Gleason system is broken down:

Lower Gleason scores, 1–4—Cells are well differentiated.

Intermediate Gleason scores, 5–7—The tumor has moderately differentiated cells.

Higher Gleason scores, 8–10—The tumor has poorly differentiated cells.

TREATMENT FOR PROSTATE CANCER

The treatment for prostate cancer may consist of no treatment (close observation), surgery, radiation therapy, hormonal therapy, chemotherapy, investigational therapy (clinical trials), or a combination of treatments. Treatment which is given to alleviate symptoms rather than cure the cancer is called palliative treatment.

In the next section, concerning treatment by stage, you'll see that there are frequently several different treatments for the same stage. Al C. is a good example. He is seventy-five years old. His wife, Mary, says he has the body and vitality of a man fifteen years younger. Al was recently diagnosed with stage B1 prostate cancer. The oncologist he saw at a major cancer center told him he was not a candidate for surgery because of his age and other medical reasons. The urologist advised against any treatment and told Al to come in every three months to be checked. Al was concerned about having no treatment. Mary was also concerned. So Al went to another urologist—who, although he treated cancer, was not at a major cancer center—for a second opinion. "He told me I should have radiation. That radiation would cure me," Al said. Then Mary said, "We don't want to make a mistake. We want to do the best thing. If radiation will cure it, shouldn't he be getting it? But the doctor at the cancer center who specializes in prostate cancer very definitely said Al should not have any treatment." They decided to make an appointment with a urologist at a different major cancer center. The third opinion might make it easier for them to decide on the treatment or it might just add to their confusion and stress. There may be no "right" decision.

The decision that a doctor makes regarding treatment is based on a number of different factors—his or her assessment of the condition of the patient, of the extent of the cancer, of the latest data available on the efficacy of the different treatment options, and of his or her own experience. Sometimes it is very obvious what the right treatment is. Other times, unfortunately, it is not, for any number of reasons. There may not have been enough time to study the long-term results of the different treatments. Or there may be two stud-

Stage A - no palpable lesion

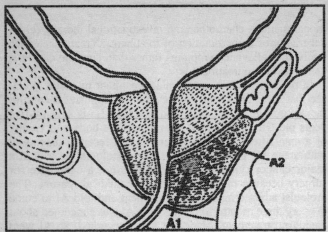

A1 - cancer cells found in only one part of the prostate
A2 - tumor cells appear in many areas of the prostate

Stage B - cancer is confined to the prostate

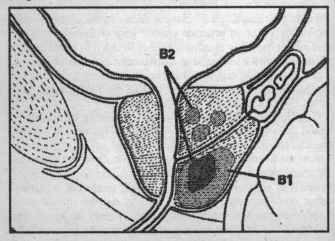

B1 - cancer very small confined to one lobe of the prostate
B2 - the cancer is more extensive and may be in both lobes

Stage C - cancer extends through the prostate capsule

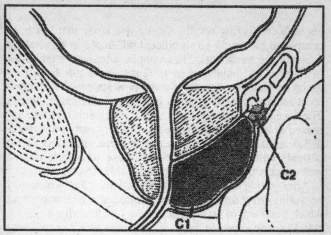

C1 - minimal extension to tissue surrounding the prostate
C2 - more extensive spread to nearby tissue

Stage D - cancer is metastatic

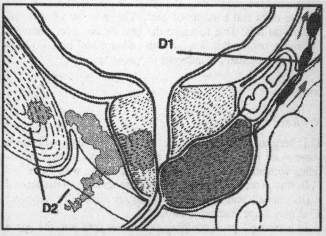

D1 - cancer has spread to distant lymph nodes
D2 - cancer has spread to bone or other distant organs

(courtesy of *Primary Care & Cancer*)

ies with conflicting results. Or the one study that has been completed has found no significant difference in survival for either of the treatments. For example, a ten-year study done in Sweden and published in 1992 suggested that for a subgroup of patients with early-stage prostate cancer, no treatment seemed to be as good as surgery or radiation treatment. The Swedish researchers reported that the survival rate appeared to be the same for patients with very early stage, well-differentiated prostate cancer who were untreated as for patients with the same stage of disease who were treated with surgery or radiation (which have side effects).

After getting different recommendations (all of which may be valid) from different experts, making a decision about which treatment to go with can be very difficult for a patient, who is *not* an expert in the field. In some cases it simply may not be possible to say which of the treatment options has the edge. What do you do if you are one of those cases and would rather not just toss a coin? You can talk with each doctor and find out why he or she prefers the treatment being recommended rather than the other treatment and then find out the risks and benefits of each. The more you know, the better you'll be able to make the best decision for yourself. For many people this is a difficult and stressful task. Following are the available treatments for prostate cancer.

Surgery

Radical Prostatectomy

This treatment is most successful with patients who have stage A or B prostate cancer. It is occasionally used on patients with stage C but is much less successful with them.

In this procedure, the entire prostate and the tissue around it (its capsule and seminal vesicles) are surgically removed. This may be performed in two ways.

In a perineal prostatectomy the doctor cuts into the space

between the scrotum and the anus, which is called the perineum. Its primary drawback is that a pelvic lymphadenectomy cannot be performed at the same time. Lymph node removal for staging requires a separate procedure. The perineal approach is a safer procedure in patients who have other medical conditions such as heart or lung disorders because it takes a shorter period of time than a retropubic prostatectomy and therefore requires less anesthesia.

In a retropubic prostatectomy the doctor cuts through the lower abdomen from the navel to the pubic bone. During this procedure the doctor can first remove the pelvic lymph nodes and examine them for cancer. If the cancer has spread to the lymph nodes, a radical prostatectomy is not done (other treatments may be used).

Anatomical Approach to Prostatectomy

This is commonly referred to as a "nerve-sparing" prostatectomy. However, Dr. Patrick Walsh, its inventor, says nerve-sparing is one aspect of the procedure, albeit, for men, usually the most significant. In the anatomical approach an assessment of the extent of the tumor is made during surgery, there is a control of blood loss, and an informed decision is made as to whether it is feasible to save one or both nerves that are necessary for erection.

The anatomical approach is a fairly new method of performing a retropubic prostatectomy. April 26, 1992, was its tenth anniversary. Dr. Walsh has now performed over a thousand radical prostatectomies. Initially he devised a technique to control bleeding and blood loss during the surgery. This enables a surgeon to cut through tissue with greater precision. Dr. Walsh then found and described the location of the nerves that are required for a normal erection of the penis. He devised a way to remove the prostate and at the same time leave those nerves intact when they do not have to be removed. Sometimes only one nerve can be spared. There are times when the nerves cannot be saved because of the extent of disease.

In the past, nearly all men undergoing a radical prostatectomy would permanently lose the ability to have an erection. *That is no longer the case!* The anatomical approach can preserve potency in a majority of patients who undergo it. Studies have found that even preserving the nerves on just one side of the prostate can preserve potency, especially in men under fifty years of age. According to Dr. Walsh, some 70 percent of the men who were potent before the surgery will eventually return to sexual functioning after the surgery. Harry L. (not his real name) had his radical prostatectomy performed by Dr. Walsh. He was in his early sixties. He says his bladder and sexual functioning kept improving as he recovered from the surgery. Following is a chart, by age and extent of surgery, from a study of 503 men, showing the recovery of sexual functioning:

Percent of Men Potent After Radical Prostatectomy

Surgical Technique	Age (years)			
	50	50–59	60–69	70
Both nerves intact	90%	82%	69%	22%
One nerve partially excised	100%	73%	50%	50%
One nerve widely excised	91%	58%	58%	-
TOTAL percent of men who retained potency after surgery	91%	75%	58%	25%

Adapted from *Prostate Cancer Update*, Johns Hopkins Medical Institutions, Volume 2, Number 1, Winter 1991.

It generally can take one to two years for potency to return as fully as possible. In some cases, there can be continued improvement for another two years. The erection may not be quite as strong as it was. The best results are obtained in younger men and men with limited disease.

Nerve-sparing can generally be performed when the tumor is small and confined to the prostate gland (stages A and B), although it may be possible in some stage C cancers. Most radical prostatectomies now performed in the United States use the anatomical approach.

For patients in whom the nerves cannot be saved, the possibility of grafting a nerve from the pelvis to restore sexual function is being investigated. Also being investigated is the possibility that a nerve growth factor (a biologically active chemical) can enhance regeneration of the nerve.

There has been some concern that sparing the nerves to preserve potency could impair the overall effectiveness of the surgery, increasing the risk of a recurrence of the cancer. Doctors agree that complete removal of the tumor is the top priority and supersedes attempts to preserve potency. According to Dr. Walsh, a group of 166 patients who underwent the nerve-sparing procedure and were kept track of for five years showed the same, or better, survival rates as men who underwent the conventional prostatectomy.

Rare side effects of a radical prostatectomy may include surgical complications, incontinence, and stricture (narrowing) of the urethra. The anatomical approach does appear to decrease the possibility of incontinence. A follow-up study of 593 patients who underwent the procedure found that 92 percent had complete urinary control. There was no patient who was totally incontinent.

Transurethral Resection of the Prostate (TURP or TUR)

TURP is generally performed in the treatment of BPH. In prostate cancer, it may be performed if the cancer is localized and very small. It may also be performed if the cancer has spread and a radical prostatectomy is not being done. In that case, it would be done as palliative treatment to relieve such symptoms as difficulty in urinating or urine retention caused by the tumor. (See the section on TURP in the chapter on benign conditions of the prostate.)

Pelvic Lymph Node Dissection

Removal of lymph nodes which may contain small metastases (cancer that has spread from the prostate) has not proven to be curative as a treatment for prostate cancer. Follow-up studies have found that a distant recurrence is likely even in patients with minimal involvement of lymph nodes. Pelvic lymph node dissection is appropriate for the staging of cancer in some patients. As noted earlier, the lymph nodes can be removed and biopsied during a retropubic prostatectomy.

Bilateral Orchiectomy

Although this is a surgical procedure, it is considered a hormonal therapy. (See hormonal therapy section in this chapter.)

Radiation Therapy

Radiation therapy is also referred to as radiotherapy, X-ray therapy, cobalt therapy, electron beam therapy, and irradiation. It uses a special kind of energy carried by waves or particles. It has been used as a treatment for cancer since the early part of the twentieth century.

Radiation can come from a machine or from a radioactive substance. It can be administered externally or internally. Radiation therapy can be used at different degrees of intensity. For example, a lung X ray uses a low level of radiation, whereas radiation for the treatment of cancer uses much higher levels. High levels of radiation can kill cells or keep them from dividing. Because most of the time cancer cells are growing and dividing more rapidly than the cells around them, radiation therapy is an effective treatment against them while doing less damage to normal cells. In addition, most normal cells seem to recover far more fully than cancer cells when exposed to radiation. Advancements in the machinery and the type of radiation used have made it more effective while at the same time reducing the number and severity of side effects.

Radiation therapy is commonly used as the primary treatment of cancer to cure the disease. It is also used as adjuvant therapy to complement another treatment, such as surgery. Radiation is also used as a palliative treatment to relieve symptoms. Both internal and external radiation are used to treat prostate cancer. Sometimes both are used.

External Radiation Therapy

This treatment uses radiation from a machine which is usually positioned a distance from the body. The radiation is directed to the site of the cancer so that healthy tissue nearby suffers minimal damage. When the radiation is used to control an area outside of the prostate to which the cancer may have spread, such as the pelvic lymph nodes, it is called extended field radiation. Curative radiation therapy in prostate cancer is generally administered five days a week for five or six weeks. Palliative radiation therapy is given for a shorter period of time.

Before treatment starts, you lie on a treatment table and a simulation is done. In a simulation the "treatment port," where the radiation will be directed, is defined by an X-ray machine and marked on the body with semipermanent ink or tiny tattoos. This generally won't take longer than an hour. When you return for the actual treatment, you get back on the table. Special shields may be put between the machine and parts of your body to help protect normal tissue and organs. Although you may be in the treatment room for around fifteen minutes, the actual treatment will be under five minutes. You have to lie still once the treatment starts so that the right target will be hit. While the treatment is taking place, the therapist will be out of the room. The therapist can always see you and can hear you as well, so you are always able to speak to the therapist. You may hear a noise while you are getting the treatment, but you will not feel any pain.

You may experience some side effects after you've undergone a number of treatments. Possible side effects are inflammation of the bowel and bladder, diarrhea, and tenesmus (the urge to defecate). These side effects can usually be managed with medication. Other possible side effects are a gradual loss of potency and infertility. If infertility is a concern, you may want to consider sperm banking. You should discuss this with your doctor. Impotence can occur one or two years after completion of the treatment. Careful treatment planning and the use of sophisticated radiation techniques such as the use of a linear accelerator can keep side effects to a minimum. Not everyone has side effects.

Internal Radiation Therapy

This therapy consists of insertion of a radioactive substance into the body in or near the cancer site to destroy it. Internal radiation places high-energy rays as close as possible to the cancer cells.

There are two types of internal radiation. In brachytherapy a radioactive source in a small sealed container is placed on the surface of the body near the tumor, a short distance from the affected area, or directly into the tissue. Brachytherapy is also known as interstitial radiation therapy and implant radiation therapy. The term *brachytherapy* is often used synonymously with *internal radiation therapy*, although it is only one specific kind of internal radiation. In intracavitary radiation the radioactive source is placed in a body cavity such as the chest. Intracavitary radiation is not used in the treatment of prostate cancer.

Brachytherapy can be used alone or in combination with external radiation therapy in the treatment of prostate cancer.

Brachytherapy affects only the prostate gland and the nearby tissue. There are several ways brachytherapy can be performed. Pellets of radiation can be implanted into the prostate either temporarily or permanently. The radioactive substances which may be used in the pellets include iodine (125I), gold (198Au), iridium (192Ir), and palladium (103Pd). Hollow steel needles filled with a radioactive substance can also be implanted into the prostate. Most of the time the insertion of the implants is done in the hospital under a general or local anesthesia. If the implant is transmitting radiation outside your body, you will probably be required to stay in a private room in the hospital. You and your implant will remain in that room until the implant is removed, which can be anywhere form one to seven days. While the implant is in place, visitors will be allowed into your room for only a short time (one to thirty minutes) and will be told to sit at least ten feet away. Most hospitals do not allow children under eighteen and pregnant women to visit patients with implants. Visits by medical staff will also be brief. Once the implant is removed, you are no longer radioactive and no longer a danger to other people.

The side effects of brachytherapy vary with the radioactive substance that is used. Some men experience no side effects. Some side effects which may occur are temporary urinary tract symptoms. A small number of men become incontinent. A very small number of men may experience impotency.

Cryosurgery

Cryosurgery is the use of extreme cold to freeze and destroy tissue. In cancer, cryosurgery is used to destroy cancer cells. Its most common use in cancer has been in the treatment of skin cancer. Cryosurgery is being investigated in the treatment of prostate cancer. It is minimally invasive. Supercooled liquid nitrogen is put in cryoprobes (needle-like instruments), which are guided by ultrasound through the skin to the site of the cancer. The cancer is frozen and destroyed. In addition, this procedure requires less hospitalization, has far fewer side effects than traditional surgery and radiation therapy, is less costly to perform, and can be done again if additional cancer is found. It is considered to be very promising by some urologists who see its primary use being in patients who cannot undergo traditional surgery of radiation; or in patients whose surgery or radiation has not been successful. Its efficacy in the treatment of prostate cancer has not yet been determined.

Hormonal Therapy

Scientists have known for years that prostate cancer cells depend on male sex hormones, known as androgens, for their growth. In 1941 it was shown that surgical removal of the testicles, which produce most of the testosterone, or administration of the female hormone estrogen to suppress the manufacture of testosterone, could cause the prostate to atrophy or decline in size.

Hormonal therapy is the use or manipulation of hormones to treat cancer. It is the mainstay of treatment for prostate cancer that has metastasized (spread) or recurred. It is the treatment of choice for stage D2 cancer which has spread to distant parts of the body, and for when the disease recurs. It may also be used in the treatment of stage D1, when the tumor is locally advanced to the regional lymph nodes.

The goal of hormonal treatment in prostate cancer is to deprive the tumor of testosterone, the predominant circulating male hormone which contributes to the tumor's growth. Hormonal therapy is not done as a cure, but rather to control the cancer and to shrink the tumor, stop it from growing, and alleviate symptoms. It can relieve pain caused by the cancer, and other symptoms such as urethral blockage by the tumor, which can make urination painful and difficult. Hormonal therapy frequently controls the cancer for prolonged periods, sometimes years.

Hormonal treatment can be performed by surgery (orchiectomy), radiation, or the administration of hormonal drugs.

Hormonal therapy using surgery is called a bilateral orchiectomy or scrotal orchiectomy. This is removal of both testicles, which are the major source of male sex hormones, particularly testosterone. It is a relatively simple and safe procedure that can be performed in the doctor's office under a local anesthesia. A small incision is made in the middle portion of the scrotum and both testicles are removed. An orchiectomy can also be performed by making two small incisions—one on each side of the scrotum. The left testicle is removed through the left opening and the right testicle through the right opening. An orchiectomy eliminates up to 95 percent of the testosterone circulating in the body. (About 5 percent of the testosterone is produced in the adrenal cortex.) It generally gives relief from symptoms quickly; however, the relief can be short-lived. The side effects of an orchiectomy are quite undesirable to many men, which is one reason some men may refuse to undergo it. The removal of both testicles results in infertility, impotency, and a loss of libido (sex drive). Another side effect can be hot flashes. This is the oldest form of hormonal therapy for prostate cancer and has been used worldwide. It is the most widely used form of hormonal therapy.

The administration of estrogens is another hormonal treatment that has also been used for years. Several forms of estrogen preparations are used, including diethylstilbestrol (DES), ethinyl estradiol, and polyestradiol. One unwelcome side effect is gynecomastia, enlargement of the breasts and breast tenderness. This can be averted by prophylactic radiation of the breasts before the start of hormonal treatment with estrogen. Prolonged treatment with estrogen may result in impotence and the loss of libido. Treatment with estrogen has also been associated with an increased risk of heart and circulatory disorders. Decreasing the dose of estrogen decreases the risk of heart problems and impotency, but the effectiveness of the therapy is also compromised. Doctors often recommend an alternative treatment for men with a history of heart problems.

The newest method of hormonal treatment for late-stage

or recurrent prostate cancer is the administration of luteinizing hormone-releasing hormone (LHRH) agonists. Two LHRH agonists in use are Lupron (leuprolide) and Zoladex (goserelin). LHRH, which is also known as gonadotropin-releasing hormone, controls the production of sex hormones in men and women. Agonists of LHRH are compounds that are structurally similar to this hormone, but instead of promoting the production of sex hormones, they suppress the production of testosterone by the testicles when given in high doses on a long-term basis.

Studies show that LHRH agonists are just as effective as estrogen therapy or orchiectomy in reducing testosterone levels in the body with fewer side effects. LHRH agonists are less likely than estrogen to cause breast enlargement or heart problems. However, as with other treatments that suppress testosterone, impotence is not uncommon and hot flashes may occur.

When LHRH agonists are used they may be accompanied by the antiandrogen flutamide (Eulexin). Flutamide was approved by the Food and Drug Administration in 1989 for use with Lupron to treat advanced prostate cancer. Flutamide blocks the effects of small amounts of male hormones produced in the adrenal glands. When flutamide is given with Lupron, it can prevent painful tumor flares, caused by a temporary increase in male hormones, which can occur during the first few weeks of treatment with LHRH agonists. Whether flutamide improves the effectiveness of androgen blockade after the first two or three months of treatment has yet to be determined.

Lupron may be given by daily injection or by depot (a pellet of the drug that is injected beneath the skin of the abdomen, where it slowly releases the drug over a month's time). Zoladex is administered only by depot.

Chemotherapy

The use of chemotherapy (anticancer) drugs in the treatment of prostate cancer has been disappointing. There has been no evidence that chemotherapy prolongs survival in men with prostate cancer. One chemotherapy drug, prednisone, may palliate, or relieve, symptoms in about a third of the cases when given in low doses. Common side effects of prednisone are stomach upset, fluid retention, and weight gain. Prednisone is taken orally.

Chemotherapy as a treatment for prostate cancer remains under investigation. Some of the drugs which have been or are in clinical trials are Adriamycin (doxorubicin), Cytoxan (cyclophosphamide), 5-FU (5-fluorouracil), Hydrea (hydroxyurea), Cisplatin, Emcyt (estramustine phosphate), methotrexate, decarbazine, and m-AMSA (amsacrine).

Clinical Trials (Investigational Treatment)

Clinical trials are the way new treatments are tested and evaluated for their efficacy in treating cancer. A clinical trial may be done to determine the most effective dose of a drug, to compare different combinations of treatments, or to determine the effect of an agent on a tumor. Many clinical trials are being performed to find new and more effective treatments for prostate cancer—and most other cancers. Clinical trials go through three phases:

- Phase I—This is the first use of the treatment on humans after animal or laboratory studies have shown it to have an effect on tumors. A Phase I trial attempts to determine whether the treatment is effective against the cancer and to find a safe and tolerable dose for humans. It is generally appropriate only for patients with widespread disease which has not responded to standard treatments. Many patients have benefitted from treatment in a Phase I trial.
- Phase II—Phase II trials attempt to determine with which other cancers the treatment may be effective.
- Phase III—In Phase III trials the new treatment is compared with the standard treatment for results and side effects. Its purpose is to determine whether the new

treatment is as good as, or better than, the standard treatment. Someone being treated in a Phase III clinical trial may very well be getting the treatment of the future.

Participation in a clinical trial is completely voluntary and you may withdraw from the trial at any time. Not everyone is eligible to take part in a clinical trial. Each study has criteria that must be met by the participant, including prior treatment, type and stage of cancer, general condition of the patient, and so forth. If you are participating in a clinical trial, you will be asked to sign an informed consent form. When you sign this form, you are saying that you know this treatment is investigational and are aware of the potential benefits and risks. Before you sign a consent form, you may want to ask the following questions:

- What is the purpose of this study?
- Who has reviewed and approved it?
- Who is sponsoring it? (Clinical trials can be sponsored by the National Cancer Institute, by the hospital, or by a pharmaceutical company.)
- What does the study involve? What kinds of tests and treatments are there?
- What is likely to happen with or without this treatment?
- What are the standard treatments and why should I go into this clinical trial instead of getting a standard treatment?
- How could this treatment affect my life on a day-to-day basis?
- What are the expected side effects?
- At this point, what kind of information is there as to the efficacy of this treatment?
- Is hospitalization required? If so, for how long and how often?
- What are the costs? Will any of the treatment be free? (Many insurance companies are not willing to reimburse patients for treatments that are investigational.)
- If the treatment is harmful or doesn't work, then what

treatment will be done?
• What type of follow-up care is part of this study?

Clinical trials being performed in the treatment of prostate cancer include alternate methods of radiation therapy, chemotherapy, and recently introduced forms of hormonal treatments using luteinizing hormone-releasing hormones (LHRH) agonists and/or antiandrogens. The status of clinical trials changes regularly—trials can become full and be accepting no new patients or the trial may be finished; new trials are added regularly. For a computer printout of the current clinical trials for your cancer, call NCI's Cancer Information Service at 1-800-4-CANCER.

Palliative Treatment

Palliative treatment is to relieve or reduce symptoms and pain. It is not done for a cure. An example of palliative treatment in prostate cancer is the use of radiation to the bone to eliminate or reduce pain in someone with metastatic cancer.

Pain and Its Management

In very early stage prostate cancer, such as A and B, there frequently is not pain (which is one of the reasons that it is hard to detect in an early stage). Pain generally ensues as the tumor gets larger and when the cancer spreads to other parts of the body, especially the bones.

A man with stage C prostate cancer may have painful urination or painful ejaculation. The enlarged tumor can block the ureters and cause pain below the ribs. Blocked blood and lymphatic vessels can cause swollen and painful legs. If nerves in the pelvic area are involved, there can be pain in that area and the pain can extend down one or both legs. The treatment for pain, at this point, is generally that used to treat what is causing the pain—the cancer. Radiation therapy is administered to the prostate to shrink it. If it is successful, the pain will decrease and eventually cease completely one or two weeks after the conclusion of the therapy. Until the radiation is effective, analgesics to suppress the pain can be taken.

Of the patients with Stage D, metastatic, cancer, 80 percent will have metastases to the bone. The ribs, spine, and long bones are most frequently involved. Patients describe the pain as a constant ache which varies in intensity. It is usually localized in one area.

Advanced prostate cancer can generate a great deal of pain. Eliminating or at least controlling it is a major component in the treatment of a patient with prostate cancer. The treatment of pain has undergone dramatic changes since the mid-1970s, when researchers discovered how opiates relieve pain and isolated natural substances in the body called endorphins and enkephalins which fight pain. New and far more effective ways of administering pain medication have been developed, as well as surgical procedures and nonmedical techniques.

If pain is managed properly, virtually no patient, cancer or otherwise, has to be in constant pain. However, many studies have shown that patients do suffer much more than they have to. They simply are not adequately treated for their pain. One reason for this is that many doctors are concerned that the patient may become addicted to the pain medication. Generally the pain is greatest when a patient is in the last stages of the disease, when addiction is not a relevant consideration. Another reason many patients are not treated correctly is that eliminating or controlling pain is a very complex procedure which frequently calls for the administration of a multitreatment approach.

Today many hospitals employ pain specialists, physicians who specialize in the treatment and management of pain. These specialists do an initial assessment of the cancer patient—to determine the source of the pain, his perception of it, and the best way to treat it in that individual patient. If their original plan is ineffective, they try other combinations. They regularly reassess the patient's response and make modifications when necessary.

Analgesics have been the mainstay of pain treatment. They do not cure the cause of the pain but suppress it temporarily. They come in three degrees of strength. Over-the-counter analgesics such as aspirin and Tylenol are the mildest. Next in strength are the nonsteroidal anti-inflammatory drugs, some of which can be bought over the counter, such as Advil, and others which require a doctor's prescription. The strongest and most effective analgesics are the narcotics, which always require a prescription. The most commonly used narcotics are morphine, codeine, Percodan (oxycodone), Levo-Dromoran (levorphanol), Dilaudid, Demerol (meperidine), methadone (Dolophine), and Numorphan (oxymorphone).

Analgesics work most quickly when injected into a vein. They are also taken by mouth, injected into a muscle, injected into subcutaneous tissue, or used as a rectal suppository. One of the newest ways of administering pain medication is the analgesic pump. The patient can turn the pump on and off and control the rate of delivery of the medication. This is commonly referred to as self-controlled analgesia (SCA) or patient-controlled analgesia (PCA). Another fairly new method of controlling pain is epidural administration, in which tiny doses of morphine are placed into the space just outside of the spinal cord.

Other methods of pain control include radiation to the specific site and surgical procedures such as pain nerve root clipping (cutting nerves high in the neck), cordotomy (cutting nerves in the spinal column), epidural dorsal column stimulator (implantation of electrodes), and rhizotomy (cutting nerves close to the spinal cord).

TREATMENT OF PROSTATE CANCER BY STAGE

The stage of the cancer is the most important information used in making a decision about the best treatment. Other factors that also can play a significant role in treatment decisions include the grade of the cells and the patient's age, physical condition, life-style, and medical history. For example, if you are over seventy and have an early-stage cancer, your doctor may recommend "expectant therapy," careful observation without treatment. Treatment will be given if and when you need it. It is not uncommon for a doctor to recommend expectant therapy. Your doctor may recommend this option because your cancer is not causing any symptoms or other problems and may be slow-growing; or because your normal life span and your life span with early-stage prostate cancer are about the same. If you are seventy-five and in great physical shape—you have the body of a sixty-five-year-old man—your doctor may advise surgery because, based on your physical condition, your life expectancy is greater.

Some patients are thrilled to hear they do not have to undergo any treatment. Other patients are very concerned. "If I have cancer and am not being treated, how will I get well?" they wonder. Or they may think the doctor is giving no treatment because they are so old is isn't worth the bother, or because it is hopeless and the treatment won't help. Whenever you have questions about your treatment, ask the doctor. And if you don't understand the answer, ask again! (See section on questions to ask in the chapter on you and your doctor.) One study comparing radical prostatectomy with just observation and treatment when needed, in men with stage A and B cancer, showed no significant difference in survival rate. However, that study, reported in 1990, included just ninety-five men. In 1992, the results of a ten-year study in Sweden found that men with early prostate cancer who were not treated for the disease had survival rates that rival those seen in men who received aggressive treatment. Additional studies are needed before any real conclusions can be drawn.

If your doctor is recommending no treatment and you are concerned, discuss it with the doctor. And if your doctor is recommending surgery and you think you may be a candidate for no treatment with regular follow-up, discuss that with your doctor.

Before making a decision on what course of treatment you

will undergo, it is always a good idea to get a second opinion. This is *not* an insult to your doctor. It does not imply that you do not trust him or her; or that you don't think he or she is competent. Getting a second opinion, especially for a disease that can be life-threatening, is a very common and accepted practice. Your doctor may even suggest that you go for a second opinion. If your doctor does not suggest getting another opinion and you would like to have one, you can ask the doctor for a referral to a doctor who specializes in prostate cancer. Another way to find a doctor for a second opinion is by calling your local medical society (it's listed in the phone book) and requesting the name of a doctor who specializes in prostate cancer. You can also call a local hospital or ask a friend who has been treated for prostate cancer or ask a friend who knows someone who has been treated. (Unfortunately, that should not be too hard to find, since prostate cancer is so prevalent.) A comprehensive cancer center is an excellent place to go for a second opinion. Comprehensive cancer centers are designated as such by the National Cancer Institute after meeting specific criteria. You'll find a list of the current institutions in the organizations appendix. As this list is updated regularly, you may want to call and make sure that the hospital is still designated as a comprehensive cancer center.

Following is the treatment by stage (the American Urological System), as recommended by the National Cancer Institute (NCI). These treatments by stage are updated by the NCI on a monthly basis whenever there is any change. This is general information and not written in stone but will give you an idea of what the treatment options are for each stage of disease. You and your doctor will decide which is the best option for you. This is the latest information available at the time of publication. To make sure that it is still current, to find out if any additional treatments have been added or studies completed, or to find out the current clinical trials that are available, call the NCI's Cancer Information Service at 1-800-4-CANCER. For a description of the treatments, see the section on treatment earlier in this chapter.

Stage A

Treatment depends on whether you have stage A1 or A2.

Stage A1

If you are older (over seventy) or have some other serious illness, you may have no treatment and just be watched closely by your doctor. If you are younger, you may have a radical prostatectomy (surgery to remove the prostate and the tissues around it).

Stage A2

Your treatment may be one of the following:

1. Careful observation without initial treatment (same as stage A1).

2. External radiation therapy. It is generally administered four to six weeks after transurethral resection to prevent stricture (an abnormal tightening) of the urethra, which can result in difficulty in urinating.

3. Radical prostatectomy with or without the nerve-sparing technique (which preserves potency) and usually with a pelvic lymph node dissection (the removal of some of the lymph nodes in the pelvis—lymph nodes are small, bean-shaped structures that are found throughout the body; they produce and store infection-fighting cells throughout the body). You may receive radiation therapy after the surgery. A radical prostatectomy may be difficult to perform if you have already had a transurethral resection of the prostate (TURP).

4. A clinical trial (a study to find a new treatment or compare different treatments to see which is most effective) of interstitial radiation therapy (implantation of radio isotopes), usually performed with a pelvic node resection. This proce-

dure may not be suitable for you if you've already had prostate surgery. Other clinical trials are also being done.

Stage B

Your treatment may be a radical prostatectomy, external radiation, or interstitial radiation.

1. If you are older or have another more serious illness, your doctor may watch you closely without treatment. Your doctor may choose this option for you because your cancer is not causing any symptoms or other problems and may be growing slowly.

2. Radical prostatectomy, usually with a pelvic lymph node dissection. You may have radiation therapy following the surgery if it is found that the tumor has penetrated the capsule surrounding the prostate or invaded the seminal vesicles or if it is found that you have a detectable level of prostate specific antigen (PSA) three weeks after the surgery. Although radiation therapy does reduce local recurrence of the cancer, it does not appear to extend survival.

3. External radiation therapy. It is generally administered four to six weeks after transurethral resection to prevent stricture of the urethra.

4. A clinical trial of internal radiation therapy, often in addition to pelvic lymph node dissection; a trial adding neutrons or protons to photon beam radiation (radiation therapy using fast-moving subatomic particles). Also being investigated is the use of ultrasound while placing radioactive sources in order to get the most effective placement.

Stage C

Your treatment may be a radical prostatectomy, external radiation, or interstitial radiation. A prostatectomy on a patient with stage C is much less effective than when it is performed on a person with stage A or B.

1. If you are older or have another more serious illness,

your doctor may follow you closely without treatment. Your doctor may choose this option for you because your cancer is not causing any symptoms or other problems and may be growing slowly.

2. Radical prostatectomy, in highly selected patients, usually with a pelvic lymph node dissection. You may have radiation therapy following the surgery if it is found that the tumor has penetrated the capsule surrounding the prostate or invaded the seminal vesicles or if it is found that you have a detectable level of prostatic specific antigen (PSA) three weeks after the surgery. Although radiation therapy does reduce local recurrence of the cancer, it does not appear to extend survival.

3. External radiation therapy. It is generally administered four to six weeks after transurethral resection to prevent stricture of the urethra.

4. A clinical trial of internal radiation therapy, often in addition to pelvic lymph node dissection; a trial adding neutrons or protons to photon beam radiation (radiation therapy using fast-moving subatomic particles).

If you are unable to have surgery or radiation therapy, your doctor may treat you to relieve symptoms such as difficulty in urinating. This is called palliative and symptomatic treatment. It may be one of the following:

1. Radiation therapy to relieve symptoms
2. Transurethral resection—surgery to cut the cancer from the prostate
3. Hormonal therapy

Stage D

The treatment chosen depends on a number of factors, including whether you have stage D1 or D2, your age, existing medical conditions, and whether the cancer has spread only to nearby lymph nodes (D1) or to other parts of the body, most often the bone (D2).

Stage D1

Your treatment may be one of the following:

1. If you are older or have another, more serious illness, your doctor may watch you closely without treatment. Your doctor may choose this option for you because your cancer is not causing any symptoms or other problems, or may be growing slowly.

2. External radiation therapy, possibly followed by hormonal therapy.

3. Clinical trials are testing new forms of radiation therapy, hormonal therapy, radical prostatectomy with an orchiectomy (surgery to remove the testicles), and radiation therapy.

Stage D2

Treatment is most often hormonal therapy. Treatment is often given to relieve symptoms such as difficulty urinating or bone pain. Your treatment may be one of the following:

1. Hormonal therapy

2. External radiation therapy to the bone to relieve symptoms

3. Transurethral resection to relieve symptoms

4. A clinical trial of chemotherapy or new forms of hormonal therapy

5. Your doctor may watch you closely and wait until you develop symptoms before giving you treatment.

Recurrent Prostate Cancer

If the cancer returns, your treatment depends on many things, including what treatment you've already had, the site of recurrence, other medical conditions, and other considerations which apply particularly to you. If you had a radical prostatectomy and the cancer comes back in only a small area, you may receive radiation therapy. If the disease has spread to other parts of the body, you will probably receive hormonal therapy. Radiation therapy may be given to relieve symptoms such as bone pain. You may also choose to take part in a clinical trial of chemotherapy or biological therapy.

Prostate Treatment and Sexual Functioning

As stated earlier, the prostate is the accessory sex gland that is responsible for producing the fluid (semen) that carries the sperm and thus plays a major role in sexual functioning. Although not all men could tell you exactly what it does, most know that their prostate gland is related to sexual functioning. Consequently, there is particular concern felt by the man who learns he has a prostate problem. Many prostate problems can be treated and cured without affecting sexual functioning. But there are times when it is affected.

INFERTILITY AND IMPOTENCY

If the prostate has been removed or is no longer able to produce semen, or the man is unable to ejaculate the semen out of his body (retrograde ejaculation), the result is infertility.

There are some treatments used for prostate problems which can result in infertility. The treatments include the following:

- TURP—surgical removal of the enlarged part of the prostate
- Open prostatectomy—surgical removal of the enlarged part of the prostate
- Radical prostatectomy—surgical removal of the entire prostate
- Bilateral orchiectomy—surgical removal of both testicles
- Hormonal therapy—administration of female hormones to eliminate testosterone; administration of LHRH agonists

Some treatments of the prostate may affect the ability to have an erection. The treatment of BPH just about never causes impotency! Ten years ago a radical prostatectomy used in the treatment of prostate cancer resulted in the inability to have an erection. Today, an anatomical approach developed in 1982 to perform a prostatectomy can preserve the nerves needed for erection and thereby prevent impotency in many patients. This is frequently referred to as nerve-sparing surgery. A bilateral orchiectomy, radiation therapy, and hormonal treatment will frequently affect the ability to have an erection, whereas removal of just one testicle rarely affects the ability to have an erection. Chemotherapy may, on rare occasions, cause a problem in getting erections. However, chemotherapy is rarely used in the treatment of prostate cancer.

There are some treatments of the prostate which may affect orgasm. A radical prostatectomy, bilateral orchiectomy, and hormonal therapy will sometimes result in a weaker orgasm. Chemotherapy may result in a weaker orgasm on very rare occasions. A transurethral resection of the prostate (TURP), a surgical procedure often used to treat an enlarged prostate, frequently results in retrograde ejaculation (dry orgasm). In retrograde ejaculation, some or all of the semen shoots back into the bladder during orgasm instead of exiting outside of the body through your penis. While the sensation felt is generally the same, infertility usually results.

SEXUAL REHABILITATION

For those men who face infertility as a result of treatment and do not want to lose the ability to father a child, sperm can be removed before the treatment and frozen for future use. The sperm is stored in a sperm bank.

There are a number of different remedies available to those men who do become impotent as a result of treatment. The most commonly used procedures are implants, external vacuum, and injections. Each treatment has advantages and disadvantages. Before making any decision on whether to undergo any treatment and which treatment to try, it is important to understand fully what can and cannot be accomplished. Getting your penis rigid will enable you to have sexual intercourse but will not solve other problems, such as low sexual desire, lack of sensation on the skin of the penis, or trouble reaching orgasm. If you are considering undergoing a surgical procedure to regain potency, you should discuss it with your wife or partner.

Following is a brief description of the different impotency treatments available.

Penile Prostheses or Implants

Surgical implant of a penile prosthesis was developed and perfected in 1960. Since then over a million men have received an implant. There are several different types of implants.

In one procedure two semirigid silicone rods are surgically

inserted into the spongy part of the penis. The penis then hangs out at about forty-five degrees from the body and stays about 80 percent erect all of the time. Urination is not affected. Sometimes the rods have a hinge so that it is easier to conceal when not in use. The rods may also have a core of wire running through them so that when you bend the penis to conceal it when you are not using it, it stays bent. By wearing athletic briefs which have heavier-than-normal elastic in front, you can usually conceal any telltale bulge at the crotch. However, it will be seen at a public urinal or locker room. Eighty to 90 percent of men with a penile implant are satisfied with their functioning during sexual intercourse. An infection can occur in 1 to 2 percent of the patients undergoing this procedure. It is very rare that there is any prolonged pain during healing or that the prosthesis will have to be repaired. The implant can be inserted under local hospitalization on an outpatient basis. If hospitalization is required, the stay may be up to four days. In 1987 the cost for a penile implant ranged from $6,000 to $10,000.

The inflatable implant was introduced in the early 1970s. You can control the penis and have it appear flaccid—the way it normally looks—or rigid, as in an erection. Two inflatable cylinders are placed in the penis. A balloon-shaped reservoir filled with salt water and X-ray dye is inserted behind the groin muscles. A small pump is placed inside the loose skin of the scrotum. In another version the pump and reservoir are combined in one piece and placed in the scrotum. When you are ready for sexual activity, you find the pump and squeeze. The fluid from the reservoir goes into the penis, stiffening it. When you no longer want the erection, you press a release valve and the fluid returns to the reservoir. With the inflatable prosthesis you generally do not have to wear any special briefs because when not in use it returns to a soft, flaccid state. Eighty to 90 percent of men are satisfied with the inflatable implants. The chance of infection while healing after the implant is about the same as that for the semirigid prosthesis—

about 1 to 2 percent. It is rare for there to be prolonged pain after healing, but there is a 5 to 15 percent chance that at some point additional surgery will be needed to repair the prosthesis. The implant can be inserted under local hospitalization on an outpatient basis. If hospitalization is required, the stay may be up to four days. In 1987 the cost for an inflatable penile implant ranged from about $10,000 to $12,000, making it a more costly procedure than the semirigid prosthesis.

Penile Injections (Intracorporeal Injections)

Medications which can produce an erection when injected into the penis have been in use since the mid-1980s. These medications are vasodilators, which means they can cause blood vessels to expand, thereby increasing blood flow. A "natural" erection is produced by the dilation of the blood vessels in the penis. The erection or dilation can last thirty minutes to two hours.

Some urologists are teaching men how to inject the medication into their penis themselves, at home. It usually takes about three office visits to learn the procedure. The use of these medications is still under investigation and long-term effects are still not clear. To minimize the risk of any side effects which may cause damage to the penis, the directions must be followed precisely. It is very important that no more than the amount of medication prescribed be used, and that it not be used more often than directed. One possible but rare side effect is an erection that does not go down. If the erection lasts four hours, the doctor should be contacted immediately. Sometimes massaging the penis or applying ice will deflate the penis. Other rare side effects include dizziness and lumps in the penis. Other, even less common side effects include bruising or bleeding at the site of injection, mild burning along the penis, difficulty in ejaculating, and swelling at the site of injection. Two medications being used are papaverine and prostaglandin (PGE-1).

External Vacuum Therapy

This is a relatively simple, mechanical way to achieve an erection without undergoing surgery. It is also relatively inexpensive, around $500. The equipment needed to perform external vacuum therapy is a clear plastic cylinder, a hand pump or battery-operated pump, and a special tension ring. To produce the erection, first the tension ring is stretched around the open end of the cylinder. Then the penis is inserted into the cylinder. The pump is then used to draw air out from the cylinder. The result is a partial vacuum around the penis, causing blood to flow into the penis and engorge it. The tension ring is then pulled off the cylinder so that it is at the base of the penis, preventing blood from leaving the penis. The cylinder is removed. The erection that is produced can last for up to half an hour with the tension ring in place.

The entire procedure takes about two minutes to achieve the erection. With a little practice, the technique is usually mastered in a short period of time. Most men find it relatively easy to do. It is a good remedy for a man who has undergone a nerve-sparing prostatectomy and whose potency is expected to eventually return.

External vacuum therapy can have some minor side effects. If the penis is kept too long under the vacuum pressure, tiny red dots may appear on the penis or it may become bruised.

Nerve Grafts/Vascular Surgery

Dr. Walsh at Johns Hopkins Medical Institution in Baltimore says that doing nerve reconstruction during a prostatectomy in men whose nerves could not be spared is being investigated and may be a viable option in the future. Replacing penile blood vessels has generally not been successful. This may be a more viable procedure as more sophisticated surgical techniques are developed.

Psychosocial Aspects
of Prostate Disease

Until now, this book has focused on the physical aspects of benign and malignant prostate disease. Both can take a psychological toll, although a diagnosis of cancer—the most serious problem—generally has the greatest emotional side effects.

Some of the issues brought up by a diagnosis of cancer are issues also raised when benign prostate disease is diagnosed, such as the realization that one has aged and may never accomplish or achieve all that was hoped for. Although this section primarily addresses the emotional impact of prostate cancer, as noted, many of these issues emerge for men with benign disease as well.

THE PSYCHOLOGICAL SIDE EFFECTS OF PROSTATE CANCER

As would be expected, the prospect of dying can be terrifying, although most men who are diagnosed with prostate cancer do not die of it. Dr. Ursula Ofman, a psychologist at Memorial Sloan-Kettering Cancer Center in New York City, works with men who have prostate cancer. She says that when men hear the words "I'm sorry, it's cancer," their first reaction is fear and panic. They are afraid they are going to die. Men with prostate cancer are not alone in this. The first concern of anyone, man or woman, diagnosed with cancer is, "I am going to die." There is also fear of intolerable pain from the cancer. The fear that cancer rouses is predictable, understandable, and normal. Prostate cancer evokes the same fears and emotions as other cancers—anxiety, guilt, anger, fear, and depression. With more understanding of the disease, many of the fears and emotions can be defused, as many of these fears are based on old myths and misconceptions. It is unfortunate that misconceptions can add additional stress and fear to an already very stressful and fearful situation.

Frequently when prostate cancer is diagnosed it can bring up midlife issues. The aging factor is right up there in plain view, since prostate cancer is a disease of older men. With the diagnosis of cancer comes the all-too-real fact of life, very prominently displayed, that one is going to die. It is frequently the first time that the man has had to face his own death on something other than a hypothetical and far-removed basis. That can bring up another issue—the fact that his life very well might end before all of the goals a man has set up for himself can be realized. This can result in feelings of regret and depression.

In addition, prostate cancer raises concerns related primarily to sexual issues. The treatment of prostate cancer can result in impotence and/or incontinence or reduced sexual and/or urinary function. The treatment that is saving your life is at the same time changing your life, perhaps irrevocably, and creating other problems.

Impotence can be a devastating side effect. To most men, the ability to function sexually, to have intercourse, is essential to their sense of manhood, their self-image. Not being able to perform sexually lowers their self-esteem and again brings up issues relating to aging and dying.

It is not unusual for a person with cancer to temporarily lose interest in sex when there is a life-threatening battle going on. The loss of interest in sex can be even greater when the cancer is affecting a sexual organ such as the prostate. Dr. Ofman says many men with prostate cancer experience a lack of sexual desire which is psychologically rather than physiologically caused. Guilt may play a role. Many people are taught as children that sex is "dirty" and not something to be enjoyed. Now they feel they are being paid back for their sexual pleasures. Some men feel like damaged goods who would be of no interest to a woman. Others will decide that they've had their share, and turn themselves off. The fear of becoming impotent as a result of the cancer or its treatment can be a self-fulfilling prophecy. The anxiety and concern over the possibility of not being able to get or sustain an erection can cause the man to be so tense that he is unable to become aroused. Once he fails to perform successfully, he worries that the same thing will happen the next time and a cycle is established.

People often feel guilty because they have cancer. They think they must have done something to deserve it. They are embarrassed at having cancer. They wrongly believe that if they had been a "good" person this would never have happened.

One of the cancer myths over the years has been that cancer is infectious and can be caught. Cancer, with a few possible rare exceptions, cannot be "caught." Nevertheless, some men are concerned that if they engage in sexual intercourse they may pass the disease on. Another fear a man may have is that sexual intercourse could be harmful to him, that perhaps it might stimulate the cancer or prompt its recurrence. Some of these same fears may be shared by the wife, who could think that she might catch cancer from her husband or that if they have sex it might affect the course of his disease and make the cancer worse.

The man with prostate cancer is not the only one affected. A diagnosis of prostate cancer also takes a toll on the people around the cancer patient, evoking many ambivalent feelings. A wife can find herself very angry that her husband has gotten this disease and is now dependent on her rather than her being dependent on him. This can evoke strong guilt feelings in the wife. "He didn't get it on purpose, it wasn't his fault," she might think. "What kind of a person am I to be angry at him when he really needs me?" This in turn can lead to more anger and resentment. Often the wife will feel that she is not being sufficiently supportive and feel guilty. She may feel angry about his lack of interest in sex and then feel guilty over her anger.

Although it's her husband who has the life-threatening illness, she too can find herself facing her own mortality for the first time, which can be very frightening. She can also feel tremendous fear and anxiety over the possibility of losing her husband and being alone, taking care of herself for the first time in many years.

There are also financial concerns, especially if limited savings are being depleted on a daily basis, money that will not be replenished if the husband dies. There is also the possibility that the wife will be left with medical bills to pay and no way to pay them. These factors can also cause resentment, fear, and guilt.

Many people are uncomfortable being around someone with cancer. They don't know what to say. They are afraid they will say the wrong thing. And they are also uncomfortable being around someone who may be dying.

Surviving cancer raises other issues and problems. Many cancer patients are surprised that, when told they are finished with treatment, they are terrified instead of being thrilled. They have been devoting energy to fighting and surviving this disease. With the treatment over, they might feel they have lost the weapons that were staving off the cancer and that now it can come back. Karrie Zampini, A.C.S.W., director of the Post-Treatment Resource Program at Memorial Sloan-Kettering Cancer Center, says, "For many people, living with the fear of recurrence and at the same time having a good quality of life is the real challenge of survivorship. Often priorities are reorganized and people have considerable clarity on what is important to them." However, the fear that the cancer will return is something that every cancer patient lives with. And although the fear does diminish, a new or familiar symptom can cause an instant return of fear, no matter how much time has passed.

TREATMENT OF PSYCHOSOCIAL PROBLEMS

Just as there are treatments to alleviate physical pain, there are techniques and treatments to relieve or decrease psychological pain. Talking with a social worker at the hospital may be helpful. The social worker or doctor may recommend counseling or psychotherapy.

Support groups are very helpful to some people. Ed Kaps had many of the typical concerns when he was diagnosed with prostate cancer. He was forty-nine when a malignant nodule was found on his prostate in 1975. Two years later he had radiation to the nodule and, as he puts it, "I thought I was home free." But that was not to be the case. In 1989 he suffered a recurrence of the prostate cancer. "I was shocked when I was told my cancer could be fatal," he says softly. His treatment was a radical prostatectomy. He desperately wanted someone to talk to—someone who was going through what he was going through. But he didn't know anyone with prostate cancer. He finally asked his doctor to send letters to other prostate cancer patients to see if any would want to get together and talk.

In 1990, Ed Kaps founded the support organization US TOO for men with prostate cancer and their family members. There was obviously a need for support groups for men with the disease. During that first year Ed Kaps received nearly eleven thousand calls from men, their wives, and other family members and friends who wanted information about the cancer and about support groups. Today he is too busy to spend much time worrying about cancer as he travels around the United States helping others set up support groups.

Ed says he was helped immediately by talking with others in the same boat. "Hearing what others were going through made my problems seem less major." There are more and more data that suggest that people who take part in support groups generally fare better. One study comparing cancer patients in support groups with others who weren't found that those in the support group scored better on psychological tests. There was a physiological difference as well. Those in the support group had a higher count of immune cells that fight tumors in their body. A ten-year follow-up in England of patients treated for advanced breast cancer found that the women who had taken part in a support group lived an average of thirty-seven months while those who hadn't taken part in a support group lived just nineteen months. Can taking part in a support group prolong your life? That is not really definitively known. However, what is known is that it can improve the quality of life for many patients.

"The first question most men have," says Ed, "is why me?" When the shock wears off, they want to know their options. After that, the most often discussed topic is impotency, followed closely by incontinence.

Dr. Ofman, who leads a support group for men with

prostate cancer, says that at first men are reluctant to speak out. But once they get involved, they are happy to have a group of people who know just what they are talking about, who have been through what they're going through.

You can ask your urologist about a prostate cancer support group. If there is not a group in the area where you live, perhaps your doctor can give you the name of a patient or two to call. If you are not comfortable with going to a support group or talking with another patient, your doctor may be able to refer you to a counselor or psychotherapist. Another resource is a social worker at the hospital.

Talking with your doctor can also help relieve some anxiety. However, that is not always so easy. Many urologists are illness oriented and are uncomfortable and shy asking a patient about sexual functioning and talking about the sexual implications of prostate cancer. Frequently the patient is older than the doctor who is treating him. This can be a source of discomfort for both the younger doctor and the older patient when it comes to discussing sexual issues. Many older patients feel that they shouldn't be concerned about sexual issues because older people shouldn't really be having sex. (I'm sure there are doctors who share this attitude.) This message is fed to us in movies and the media on a fairly regular basis. Men who have bought into that—and many have—will find it very difficult if not impossible to bring up sexual issues. Most of the men being diagnosed with prostate cancer are still of the generation that was not as open and free speaking about sex as young and middle-aged people are today. If the patient doesn't bring it up, the doctor doesn't bring it up—and vice versa. If you have a doctor who doesn't say anything about sexual issues and you have concerns, as difficult as you may find it you will have to broach the subject. If the issues are not discussed, your doctor won't be affected—but you very well may be.

Ed Kaps says too often the problems that other family members are having are ignored. The US TOO support groups are open to wives and other family members and friends of the patient. Sometimes just the wives meet without their husbands. "The importance of open and honest communication between the patient and the people who are going through it with him," says Ed, "cannot be stressed enough. If people can express their fears and anxieties, there is more possibility for greater understanding and support." A support group and/or counseling may be helpful for family members.

There are other techniques that can be used to alleviate or reduce stress. One is imagery, which is also referred to as visualization. It is a mind exercise in which you create a picture in the mind, like a daydream. (This can also be used to control pain and fight the cancer.) Another method is relaxation, which can be done in a number of different ways. And yet another technique which may be helpful is biofeedback, in which you learn to control the body's automatic functions, such as blood pressure and muscle tension.

There is no question that tremendous progress has been made in the detection, diagnosis, and treatment (medical and psychological) of both benign and malignant disease of the prostate as well as some of the side effects of various treatments. Physicians and researchers can only do so much. Your own participation in your health care is a vital component. *The Prostate Answer Book* was written to help you do that.

APPENDIX I:
ORGANIZATIONS

AMC Cancer Research Center—Denver, Colorado; its toll-free number, 1-800-525-3777, is available 8:30 A.M. to 5:00 P.M., Mountain Time. Information is provided on the causes, prevention, detection, diagnosis, and treatment of cancer, as well as treatment facilities and rehabilitation and counseling services.

American Association of Tissue Banks—1350 Beverly Road, Suite 220A, McLean, Virginia 22101; (703)827-9582. This organization can tell you where you can find a sperm bank facility in your area.

American Cancer Society (ACS)—1599 Clifton Road NE, Atlanta, Georgia; (404)320-3333; the toll-free cancer response line is 1-800-ACS-2345 and is in operation from 8:30 A.M. to 4:30 P.M. ACS is a nationwide voluntary health organization. It supports and funds research; provides education on cancer prevention, early detection, and treatment; provides services for cancer patients and their families; and provides free literature, including the pamphlet *Facts on Prostate Cancer*. There are fifty-seven chartered divisions and about three thousand local units. Following are the chartered divisions by state:

Alabama—505 Brookwood Boulevard, Homewood AL 35209; (205)879-2242

Alaska—406 West Fireweed Lane, Anchorage, AK 99503; (907)277-8696

Arizona—2929 East Thomas Road, Phoenix, AZ 85016; (602)224-0524

Arkansas—901 N. University, Little Rock, AR 72207; (501)664-3480

California—1710 Webster Street, P.O. Box 2061, Oakland, CA 94612; (510)893-7900

Colorado—2255 South Oneida, P.O. Box 24669, Denver, CO 80224; (303)758-2030

Connecticut—Barnes Park South, 14 Village Lane, Wallingford, CT 06492; (203)265-7161

Delaware—92 Read's Way, New Castle, DE 19720; (302)324-4227

District of Columbia—1825 Connecticut Avenue, Washington, DC 20009; (202)483-2600

Florida—1001 S. MacDill Avenue, Tampa, FL 33629; (813)253-0541

Georgia—46 Fifth Street NE, Atlanta, GA, 30308; (404)892-0026

Hawaii—Community Services Center Building, 200 N. Vineyard Boulevard, Honolulu, HI 96817; (808)531-1662

Idaho—2676 Vista Avenue, P.O. Box 5386, Boise, ID 83705; (208)343-4609

Illinois—77 E. Monroe, Chicago, IL 60603; (312)641-6150

Indiana—8730 Commerce Park Place, Indianapolis, IN 46268; (317)872-4432

Iowa—8364 Hickman Road, Suite D, Des Moines, IA 50325; (515)253-0147

Kansas—1315 SW Arrowhead Road, Topeka, KS 66604; (913)273-4114

Kentucky—701 W. Muhammad Ali Boulevard, Louisville, KY 40201-1807; (502)584-6782

Louisiana—Fidelity Homestead Building, 837 Gravier Street, Suite 700, New Orleans, LA 70112-1509; (504)523-2092

Maine—52 Federal Street, Brunswick, ME 04011; (207)729-2339

Maryland—8219 Town Center Drive, White Marsh, MD 21162-0082; (410)931-6868

Massachusetts—247 Commonwealth Avenue, Boston, MA 02116; (617)267-2650

Michigan—1205 E. Saginaw Street, Lansing, MI 48906; (517)371-2920

Minnesota—3316 W. 66th Street, Minneapolis, MN 55435; (612)925-2772

Mississippi—1380 Livingston Lane, Lakeover Office Park, Jackson, MS 39213; (601)362-8874

Missouri—3322 American Avenue, Jefferson City, MO 65102; (314)893-4800

Montana—313 N. 32nd Street, Suite #1, Billings, MT 59101; (406)252-7111

Nebraska—8502 W. Center Road, Omaha, NE 68124-5255; (402)393-5800

Nevada—1325 E. Harmon, Las Vegas, NV 89119; (702)798-6857

New Hampshire—360 Route 101, Unit 501, Bedford, NH 03102-6800; (603)472-8899

New Jersey—2600 Route 1, CN 2201, North Brunswick, NJ 08902; (908)297-8000

New York—6725 Lyons Street, P.O. Box 7, East Syracuse, NY 13057; (315)437-7025

- Long Island—75 Davids Drive, Hauppauge, NY 11788; (516)436-7070
- New York City—19 W. 56th Street, New York, NY 10019; (212)586-8700
- Queens—112-25 Queens Boulevard, Forest Hills, NY 11375; (718)263-2224
- Westchester—30 Glenn Street, White Plains, NY 10603; (914)949-4800

North Carolina—11 S. Boylan Avenue, Suite 221, Raleigh, NC 27603; (919)834-8463

North Dakota—123 Roberts Street, P.O. Box 426, Fargo, ND 58107; (701)232-1385

Ohio—5555 Frantz Road, Dublin, OH 43017; (614)889-9565

Oklahoma—3000 United Founders Boulevard, Suite 136, Oklahoma City, OK 73112; (405)843-9888

Oregon—0330 SW Curry, Portland, OR 97201; (503)295-6422

Pennsylvania—P.O. Box 897, Route 442 & Sipe Avenue, Hershey, PA 17033-0897; (717)533-6144

- Philadelphia—1422 Chestnut Street, Philadelphia, PA 19102; (215)665-2900

Puerto Rico—Calle Alverio #577, Esquina Sargento Medina, Hato Rey, PR 00918; (809)764-2295

Rhode Island—400 Main Street, Pawtucket, RI 02860; (401)722-8480

South Carolina—128 Stonemark Lane, Columbia, SC 29210; (803)750-1693

South Dakota—4101 Carnegie Place, Sioux Falls, SD 57106-2322; (605)361-8277

Tennessee—1315 Eighth Avenue South, Nashville, TN 37203; (615)255-1227

Texas—2433 Ridgepoint Drive, Austin, TX 78754; (512)928-2262

Utah—610 East South Temple, Salt Lake City, UT 84102; (801)322-0431

Vermont—13 Loomis St., P.O. Box 1452, Montpelier, VT 05601-1452; (802)223-2348

Virginia—4240 Park Place Court, Glen Allen, VA 23060; (804)270-0142 or 1-800-ACS-2345

Washington—2120 First Avenue North, Seattle, WA 98109-1140; (206)283-1152

West Virginia—2428 Kanawha Boulevard East, Charleston, WV 25311; (304)344-3611

Wisconsin—615 N. Sherman Avenue, Madison, WI 53704; (608)249-0487

Wyoming—2222 House Avenue, Cheyenne, WY 82001; (307)638-3331

American Fertility Society—1209 Montgomery Highway, Birmingham, Alabama 35216-2809; (205)978-5000. Printed information is available on sperm banking and local facilities.

American Foundation for Urologic Disease, Inc.—1120 North Charles Street, Suite 401, Baltimore, Maryland 21201; its toll-free number is 1-800-242-2383. It has the following free pamphlets available: *Prostate Disease: Vital Information for Men Over 40; Prostate Cancer: What Every Man Should Know; Enlarged Prostate: BPH and Male Urinary Problems;* and *Prostatitis: Answers to Your Questions.*

American Medical Association—515 North State Street, Chicago, Illinois 60610; (312)464-5000. Can provide information on a doctor—when he or she was licensed, his or her specialty, if he or she is board certified. (The *Directory of Medical Specialists* lists the qualifications of medical doctors and should be available in medical libraries and the public library.)

Biogenics Corporation—1130 Route 22 West, P.O. Box 1290, Mountainside, New Jersey 07092; 1-800-942-4646; (201)399-8228. A facility which banks sperm.

Board Certification—1-800-776-2378. Can provide information on whether a doctor is board certified. (The *Directory of*

Medical Specialists lists the qualifications of medical doctors and should be available in medical libraries and the public library.)

Cancer Care—1180 Avenue of the Americas, New York, New York 10036; (212)221-3300. A nonprofit social service agency. Helps patients and family members cope with the emotional and financial consequences of cancer. It generally serves the New York metropolitan area but responds to phone calls and letters from all over the United States, providing information and referrals whenever possible.

Cancer Information Service (CIS)—the nationwide toll-free 1-800-4-CANCER number is available 9:00 A.M. to 10:00 P.M. weekdays and 10:00 A.M. to 6:00 P.M. Saturday. Funded largely by the National Cancer Institute. Information specialists can tell callers the latest state-of-the-art treatment for a particular cancer, where clinical trials are taking place, and can provide information about detection, prevention, diagnosis, and support groups. Free NCI booklets are available, including *What You Need to Know About Prostate Cancer*.

CanSurmount—a program sponsored by the American Cancer Society (ACS) which provides a short-term visitor program for cancer patients and family members in the hospital and/or at the home for support and encouragement; for information contact your local ACS or call 1-800-ACS-2345.

Chemotherapy Foundation—183 Madison Avenue, Suite 403, New York, New York 10016; (212)213-9292. Has free publications available.

Concern for the Dying—250 West 57th Street, New York, New York 10107; (212)246-6962. A nonprofit educational council advocating the patient's right to take part in decisions regarding treatment and life-sustaining measures. Provides information on the "living will"; current laws in each state on euthanasia, death, and dying; psychological and legal counseling; and referral to local organizations for other types of assistance.

Consumer Product Safety Commission (CPSC)—Washington, DC 20207; 1-800-638-CPSC. Has free pamphlets.

Corporate Angel Network (CAN)—Westchester County Airport, Building 1, White Plains, New York 10604; (914)328-1313. Nonprofit organization that finds available space on corporate jets for cancer patients in need of transportation for treatment, consultations, or checkups. The service is free for the patient and one attendant or family member.

Environmental Protection Agency (EPA)—4001 M Street, Washington, DC 20460; (202)829-3535. Has information on environmental factors which may play a role in cancer.

Food and Drug Administration (FDA)—(HFE-88), 5600 Fishers Lane, Rockville, Maryland 20857; (301)245-8012. Gives approval for the sale of over-the-counter and prescription drugs. Regulates medical devices. Can give information on whether a drug has been approved.

Geddings Osbon Foundation—1246 Jones Street, Augusta, Georgia 30901; 1-800-433-4215. Does research and public education on impotency. Has free, comprehensive booklet called *Impotence: Current Diagnosis and Treatment*.

Help for Incontinence (HIP)—Simon Foundation for Continence, P.O. Box 544, Union, South Carolina 29379; 1-800-237-4666 8:00 A.M. to 5:00 P.M. Will send informational package.

Hereditary Cancer Institute—Henry Lynch, M.D., Creighton University School of Medicine, California at 24th, Omaha, Nebraska 68178; (402)280-2942. Provides free cancer-risk information and other forms of genetic counseling.

HospiceLink—Hospice Education Institute, Five Essex

Square, Suite 3-B, P.O. Box 713, Essex, Connecticut 06426-0713; 1-800-331-1620; in Alaska and Connecticut, (203)767-1620. A nonprofit service which has information about hospice care. Can provide cancer patients and their families with referrals to local hospice programs and publications.

I Can Cope—A patient education program of the American Cancer Society (ACS) designed to help patients, families, and friends cope with the day-to-day issues of living with cancer. An eight-session course taught by health professionals from the hospital and community is usually offered through the local hospital. For information on this program, contact the ACS.

Impotence Hotline—The Impotence Information Center, P.O. Box 9, Minneapolis, Minnesota 55440; 1-800-843-4315. Will send general information and make physician referrals.

Impotence Institute International—87-119 South Ruth Street, Maryville, Tennessee 37801-5764. Publishes a newsletter for men with impotency problems.

Make Today Count—101½ South Union Street, Alexandria, Virginia 22314-3323; (703)548-9714 or (703)548-9674. Patients with cancer or other life-threatening illnesses and their families are brought together for a self-help approach to coping with a serious illness. There are over two hundred chapters in the United States, Canada, and Europe.

National Center for Nutrition and Dietetics—216 West Jackson Boulevard, Suite 8, Chicago, Illinois 60606-695; its toll-free Consumer Nutrition Hotline is 1-800-366-1655. Registered dietician available 9:00 A.M. to 4:00 P.M. Central Time; pamphlets available on topics such as fiber, low fat, and vitamins.

National Coalition for Cancer Survivorship—1010 Wayne Avenue, 5th Floor, Silver Spring, Maryland 20910; (301)585-2616. A network of independent groups and individuals offering support to cancer survivors, family members, and friends. Provides information and resources on support and life after a cancer diagnosis.

National Hospice Organization—1901 North Moore Street, Suite 901, Arlington, Virginia 22209; (703)243-5900. An Association of groups that provide hospice care. Founded in 1978 to promote and maintain quality hospice care and encourage support for patients and family members. Can provide information on local hospices.

National Institute of Diabetes and Digestive and Kidney Diseases (NIDDK)—Founded in 1950 by Congress, it is part of the National Institutes of Health (NIH). It conducts research in disorders of the lower urinary tract, including BPH and prostatitis. For the free booklet *Prostate Enlargement: Benign Prostatic Hyperplasia,* write to the National Kidney and Urologic Diseases Information Clearinghouse, Box NKU-DIC, 9000 Rockville Pike, Bethesda, Maryland 20892. The NIDDK has established six new research centers. There are two that deal with prostate problems:

John T. Grayhack, M.D. (prostate enlargement)
Department of Urology
Northwestern University Medical School
303 East Chicago Avenue
Chicago, Illinois 60611
(312)908-8145

Ahmad Elbadawi, M.D. (urinary tract obstruction)
SUNY Upstate Center
750 East Adams Street
Syracuse, New York 13210
(315)464-5737

National Prostate Cancer Detection Project (NPCDP)—A group of institutions in the United States and Canada which are working together to set a standard of screening for prostate cancer. Approximately five thousand men aged fifty-five to seventy, with no known risk for prostate cancer, will be screened and followed for five years. All the institutions participating will use the same equipment. The men will be screened yearly with transrectal ultrasound, digital rectal exam, and prostate-specific antigen (PSA). The following institutions are taking part in the study:

- Cook County Hospital, Chicago, Illinois
- Long Beach Memorial Medical Center, University of California at Irvine, Long Beach, California
- MD Anderson Cancer Center, University of Texas, Houston, Texas
- New England Deaconess Hospital, Harvard University, Boston, Massachusetts
- Northwest Regional Center, Urology Clinic of Yakima, Yakima, Washington
- The Ohio State University, University Hospitals, Columbus, Ohio
- Catherine McAuley Health Center, Saint Joseph Mercy Hospital, Ann Arbor, Michigan
- Saint Joseph's Hospital, Terry Fox Memorial Early Prostate Cancer Detection Clinic, Saint John, New Brunswick
- Toronto General Hospital, University of Toronto, Toronto, Ontario
- Urologic Consultants, Saint Vincent Medical Office, Portland, Oregon

Patient Advocates for Advanced Cancer Treatment (PAACT)—P.O. Box 1656, Grand Rapids, Michigan 49501; (616)453-1477; fax (616)453-1846. Nonprofit organization which has information for patients with advanced disease. Publishes a newsletter and yearly *Prostate Cancer Report*.

Society for the Right to Die—250 West 57th Street, New York, New York 10107; (212)246-6973. Nonprofit organization that provides information and a copy of a "living will" upon request. Promotes right-to-die legislation and citizens' rights.

US TOO, P.O. Box 7173, Oakbrook Terrace, Illinois 60181; 1-800-828-7866, or (708)627-6834 in Chicago area. A support group for prostate cancer survivors and those diagnosed with prostate cancer. Information, counseling, and educational meetings are held, as well as monthly support meetings for prostate patients and their families. Sponsored by the American Foundation for Urologic Disease.

APPENDIX II: COMPREHENSIVE CANCER CENTERS

Comprehensive Cancer Centers are designated by the National Cancer Institute (NCI). To be so designated, an institution must first secure a peer-reviewed cancer center support grant from the NCI. Then a review committee made of nonfederal scientists determines if the centers meet the set criteria. The latest criteria, as of 1989, are:

1. Must have a strong core of basic laboratory research in several fields.

2. Must have ways to transfer research findings into clinical practice.

3. Must conduct clinical trials, especially ones of importance to the community served by the center.

4. Must participate in high-priority clinical trials.

5. Must conduct research in the areas of cancer prevention and control.

6. Must provide research training and continuing education for health care professionals.

7. Must offer a wide range of cancer information services for patients, health professionals, and the surrounding community.

8. Must provide community service and outreach activities related to cancer prevention and control.

Following are the NCI-designated comprehensive cancer centers, by state as of 1993:

ALABAMA—University of Alabama Comprehensive Cancer Center, 1918 University Boulevard, Basic Health Sciences Building, Room 108, Birmingham, AL; (205)934-6612

ARIZONA—University of Arizona Cancer Center, 1501 North Campbell Avenue, Tucson, AZ 85724; (602)626-6372

CALIFORNIA—The Kenneth Norris, Jr., Comprehensive Cancer Center, University of Southern California, 1441 Eastlake Avenue, Los Angeles, CA 90033-0804; (213)226-2370

Jonsson Comprehensive Cancer Center, University of California at Los Angeles, 200 Medical Plaza, Los Angeles, CA 90027; (213)206-0278

CONNECTICUT—Yale University Comprehensive Cancer Center, 333 Cedar Street, New Haven, CT 06510; (203)785-6338

DISTRICT OF COLUMBIA—Lombardi Cancer Research Center, Georgetown University Medical Center, 3800 Reservoir Road NW, Washington, D.C. 20007; (202)687-2192

FLORIDA—Sylvester Comprehensive Cancer Center, University of Miami Medical School, 1475 Northwest 12th Avenue, Miami, FL 33136; (305)548-4800

MARYLAND—The Johns Hopkins Oncology Center, 600 North Wolfe Street, Baltimore, MD 21205; (301)955-8638

MASSACHUSETTS—Dana-Farber Cancer Institute, 44 Binney Street, Boston, MA 02115; (617)732-3214

MICHIGAN—Meyer L. Prentis Comprehensive Cancer Center of Metropolitan Detroit, 110 East Warren Avenue, Detroit, MI 48201; (313)745-4329

University of Michigan Cancer Center, 101 Simpson Drive, Ann Arbor, MI 48109-0752; (313)936-9583

MINNESOTA—Mayo Comprehensive Cancer Center, 200 First Street Southwest, Rochester, MN 55905; (507)284-3413

NEW HAMPSHIRE—Norris Cotton Cancer Center, Dartmouth-Hitchcock Medical Center, 2 Maynard Street, Hanover, NH 03756; (603)646-5505

NEW YORK—Memorial Sloan-Kettering Cancer Center, 1275 York Avenue, New York, New York 10021; 1-800-525-2225

Kaplan Cancer Center—New York University Medical Center, 1462 First Avenue, New York, New York 10016-91003; (212)263-6485

Roswell Park Cancer Institute—Elm and Carlton Streets, Buffalo, New York 14263; (716)845-4400

NORTH CAROLINA—Duke Comprehensive Cancer Center, P.O. Box 3814, Durham, North Carolina 27710; (919)286-5515

Lineberger Comprehensive Cancer Center, University of North Carolina School of Medicine, Chapel Hill, North Carolina 27599; (919)966-4431

Cancer Center of Wake Forest University at the Bowman Gray School of Medicine, 300 South Hawthorne Road, Winston-Salem, North Carolina 27103; (919)748-4354

OHIO—Ohio State University Comprehensive Cancer Center, 410 West 10th Avenue, Columbus, Ohio 43210; (614)293-8619

PENNSYLVANIA—Fox Chase Cancer Center, 7701 Burholme Avenue, Philadelphia, Pennsylvania 19111; (215)728-2570

University of Pennsylvania Cancer Center, 3400 Spruce Street, Philadelphia, Pennsylvania 19104; (215)662-6364

Pittsburgh Cancer Institute, 200 Meyran Avenue, Pittsburgh, Pennsylvania 15213-2592; 1-800-537-4063

TEXAS—The University of Texas M. D. Anderson Cancer Center, 1515 Holcombe Boulevard, Houston, Texas 77030; (713)792-3245

VERMONT—Vermont Cancer Center, University of Vermont, 1 South Prospect Street, Burlington, Vermont 05401; (804)656-4580

WASHINGTON—Fred Hutchinson Cancer Research Center, 1124 Columbia Street, Seattle, Washington 98104; (206)467-4675

WISCONSIN—Wisconsin Clinical Cancer Center, University of Wisconsin, 600 Highland Avenue, Madison, Wisconsin 53792; (608)263-8090

BIBLIOGRAPHY

Berger, Richard E., and Deborah Berger. *BioPotency: A Medical Guide to Sexual Success*. Emmaus, PA: Rodale Press, 1986. (Facts on erection problems and their treatment.)

Facts on Prostate Cancer. (Free American Cancer Society pamphlet available by calling 1-800-ACS-2345.)

Graham, Jory. *In the Company of Others: Understanding the Human Needs of Cancer Patients*. New York: Harcourt Brace Jovanovich, 1987. (Patients' rights, emotions, sex, and other cancer-related issues.)

Holleb, Arthur, ed. *The American Cancer Society Cancer Book: Prevention, Detection, Diagnosis, Treatment, Rehabilitation, Cure*. New York: Doubleday, 1986. (Reference guide on different types of cancer.)

Kilman, Peter, and Katherine Mills. *All About Sex Therapy*. New York: Plenum, 1983. (Guide to seeking help for sexual problems.)

Kushner, Harold. *When Bad Things Happen to Good People.* New York: Avon, 1983. (Discussion of guilt, blame, and other reactions of cancer patients and family members.)

LeShan, Lawrence. *You Can Fight for Your Life.* New York: M. Evans, 1977. (Emotional aspects of cancer.)

LeShan, Lawrence. *Cancer as a Turning Point: A Handbook for People with Cancer, Their Families and Health Professionals.* New York: Dutton, 1989. (Mobilizing the patient's healing abilities through the involvement of family and professionals.)

Morra, Marion, and Eve Potts. *Choices: Realistic Alternatives in Cancer Treatment.* New York: Avon, revised 1994. (Information about cancer in a question-and-answer format.)

Prostate Cancer: What Everyone Should Know. (Free pamphlet available by writing to TAP Pharmaceutical, Inc., Bannockburn Lake Office Plaza, 2355 Waukegan Road, Deerfield, IL 60015.)

Prostate Disease: Vital Information for Men Over 40; Prostate Cancer: What Every Man Should Know; Enlarged Prostate: BPH and Male Urinary Problems; and *Prostatitis: Answers to Your Questions.* (Available from the American Foundation for Urologic Disease by calling 1-800-242-2383.)

Prostate Enlargement: Benign Prostatic Hyperplasia. (Free pamphlet available by writing to the National Kidney and Urologic Diseases Information Clearinghouse, Box NKUDIC, 9000 Rockville Pike, Bethesda, MD 20892.)

Radiation Therapy and You: A Guide to Self-Help During Treatment. (Available free from the National Cancer Institute by calling 1-800-4-CANCER.)

Schover, Leslie. *Prime Time: Sexual Health for Men over Fifty.* New York: Holt, Rinehart & Winston, 1984. (Facts on sex and aging, hormone therapy, choosing a penile prosthesis, sex therapy, and sexual communication.)

Schover, Leslie. *Sexuality and Cancer: For the Man Who*

Has Cancer, and His Partner. Atlanta: American Cancer Society, 1988. (Free booklet available by calling 1-800-ACS-2345.)

Siegel, Bernie. *Love, Medicine and Miracles*. New York: Harper & Row, 1986. (Former surgeon's experience with self-healing by cancer patients.)

Simonton, O. C., S. Mathers-Simonton, S., and J. Creighton. *Getting Well Again*. New York: Bantam Books, 1980. (Medicine, visual imagery, exercise, relaxation, and psychotherapy for cancer patients.)

Taking Time: Support for People with Cancer and the People Who Care About Them. (Available free from the National Cancer Institute by calling 1-800-4-CANCER.)

What You Need to Know About Prostate Cancer (Available free from the National Cancer Institute by calling 1-800-4-CANCER.)

Zilbergeld, Bernie. *Male Sexuality: A Guide to Sexual Fulfillment*. New York: Bantam Books, 1978. (Myths of male sexuality, self-help programs for premature ejaculation and erection problems.)

GLOSSARY

abdomen—the part of the body below the diaphragm and between the chest and pelvis.

acid phosphatase test—the examination of blood for the presence of an enzyme secreted by the prostate gland. This may be done in the diagnosis of prostate cancer and other disorders of the prostate.

acute—rapidly developing, quick, sudden.

acute bacterial prostatitis (acute infectious prostatitis)—an infection in the prostate gland which comes on suddenly.

acute urinary retention—the sudden inability to urinate.

adenocarcinoma—a cancer made up of abnormal gland (*adeno* means "gland") cells that arise from the lining or inner surface of an organ. It can develop in virtually any part of the body. More than 95 percent of prostate cancers are adenocarcinomas.

adjuvant therapy—a treatment used in addition to the primary treatment. When it is used before the primary treatment it is called neoadjuvant treatment.

adrenal glands—a pair of small organs right above the kidneys. They produce hormones, including androgens.

alkaline phosphatase—an enzyme produced mainly by the liver and bone.

androgen hormone—any hormone that produces male physical characteristics, such as facial hair or deep voice. The main androgen is testosterone.

anesthesia—a state of total or partial loss of consciousness and sensation induced in a patient to allow a surgical or painful procedure to be performed. It can be topical (administered directly to area involved), local (confined to one part of the body), or general (a total loss of consciousness).

antiandrogen drug—a substance that blocks the activity of an androgen hormone.

anticancer drug—a substance that attacks cancer cells; chemotherapy.

anus—the opening at the lower end of the large intestine through which body waste passes.

artificial urinary sphincter—a prosthesis used to restore control of the bladder in an incontinent person by constricting the bladder.

aspiration—withdrawal of fluid from the body by use of suction.

bacteria—one-celled organisms which may cause disease (infection or inflammation) in the body.

bacteriuria—the presence of bacteria in the urine.

benign prostatic hyperplasia (BPH)—enlargement of the prostate caused by an abnormal growth of the number of cells. This is a benign (noncancerous) condition. Benign prostatic hyperplasia and benign prostatic hypertrophy are frequently used interchangeably.

benign prostatic hypertrophy (BPH)—enlargement of the prostate caused by an enlargement of the cells that make up the prostate. The prostate pushes against the urethra and bladder, blocking the flow of urine. This is a noncancerous condition. Benign prostatic hypertrophy and benign prostatic hyperplasia are frequently used interchangeably.

benign tumor—a mass in the body which does not invade and destroy the tissue in the body where it originated and does not spread to distant sites. A benign tumor is noncancerous, not malignant.

biopsy—the microscopic examination of tissue cells removed from the body to determine if cancer cells are present. In prostate cancer, a biopsy is the only way to confirm a diagnosis of cancer.

biopty gun—the newest, "high tech" method of performing a prostate biopsy. It uses a needle in a spring-loaded "gun" to obtain tissue for a biopsy.

bladder—the organ in the body that stores urine.

bladder catheterization—passage of a catheter (narrow, flexible tube) into the bladder.

bladder neck contracture—an abnormal narrowing of the bladder neck so that it is difficult for urine to pass through.

bladder outlet—the first part of the bladder through which urine flows when it leaves the bladder.

blood urea nitrogen (BUN)—a blood test to measure kidney function.

bone scan—a two-dimensional image taken of the entire body skeleton or specific area after the injection of a radioactive tracer substance into the blood, which carries it to the bone.

brachytherapy—treatment with a radioactive source placed in or near the cancer in the prostate. Sometimes this term is used instead of *internal radiation therapy*. It is one type of internal radiation therapy.

cancer—a general term for over a hundred diseases characterized by the uncontrolled, abnormal growth of cells. Cancer cells can be spread to other parts of the body through the bloodstream and lymphatic system.

capsule—the structure in which something is enclosed. The prostate gland is contained in a capsule.

carcinoma—one of five basic types of cancer. It starts in the tissues that line or cover an organ. Carcinomas account for 80 to 90 percent of all cancers. The word *carcinoma* is frequently used synonymously with cancer.

CAT (computerized axial tomography) scan (computed tomography CT scan)—a diagnostic procedure combining an X ray with a computer to produce highly detailed cross-sectional pictures of a part of the body or the whole body.

catheter—a soft lubricated tube. A catheter may be used to drain urine from the bladder.

cells—the basic structural and functional units of the body.

chemotherapy—treatment or control of cancer with anticancer drugs. Chemotherapy may be used before surgery to shrink the tumor, or instead of surgery. Chemotherapy is commonly referred to as chemo.

chlamydia—a family of bacterial organisms that commonly cause infection in the urethra as well as other parts of the body.

chronic—continuous or of long duration. Cancer is commonly referred to as a chronic disease because many people live with the disease for many years.

chronic bacterial prostatitis (chronic infectious prostatitis)—an infection in the prostate gland that persists over a long period of time.

clinical trials (investigational trials)—a systematic evaluation of a possible new cancer treatment with cancer patients. Each study is designed to answer specific questions about the treatment.

cobalt—a radioactive material that may be used in external radiation therapy. It is usually used in supervoltage machines which deliver radiation to the tumor site without affecting the skin.

cobalt 60—a supervoltage machine used to disseminate radiation in external radiation therapy.

creatinine—a substance excreted by the kidneys. Its level in the blood can provide information about the kidneys' functioning.

core-needle biopsy (needle biopsy, wide-core needle biopsy, or punch biopsy)—A special needle which contains a minuscule cutting instrument is used in the removal of tissue in order to perform microscopic examination for cancer cells.

cryosurgery—the use of extreme cold to freeze and destroy diseased tissue in a specific part of the body.

cystitis—an infection of the bladder frequently characterized by a frequent urge to urinate, a painful, burning sensation during urination, and sometimes, the passage of blood in the urine.

cystoscopy—a visual examination of the bladder using a cystoscope, a lighted, tubular instrument.

decompensated bladder—a condition in which the organ of the body which stores urine retains some after urination instead of emptying completely.

diagnosis—the process of determining the nature of disease so that treatment can be administered.

digital rectal exam (DRE)—a common screening procedure for prostate disease, including cancer. A doctor inserts a finger into the rectum to feel the size and shape of the prostate through the wall of the rectum.

dosimetrist—a person trained to plan and calculate the proper radiation dose for treatment.

DRE—*see* DIGITAL RECTAL EXAM.

ejaculation—ejection of sperm and seminal fluid through the penis to the outside of the body.

epithelium—the tissue that covers the external and internal surfaces of the body, including the lining of vessels and small cavities.

erectile dysfunction—*see* IMPOTENCE.

estrogen—female sex hormones that are responsible for the development of secondary sex characteristics such as the growth of breasts. Synthetic estrogens may be used in the treatment of prostate cancer.

excretory urogram—*see* INTRAVENOUS PYELOGRAM.

external radiation therapy (teletherapy)—a treatment using high-energy radiation therapy from a machine located outside of the body. The radiation therapy is usually directed at a specific body site. Approximately 50 percent of all cancer patients receive radiation therapy.

external urethral sphincter—a donut-shaped muscle that can voluntarily constrict the passage of urine from the bladder.

external vacuum therapy—a noninvasive mechanical procedure to produce a temporary erection.

false negative—a term that refers to the results of a test which incorrectly report there is no disease present.

false positive—a term that refers to the results of a test which incorrectly report there is disease present.

fine-needle aspiration—the use of a thin needle to withdraw cells or tissue from a suspicious area in the body. The tissue is then biopsied (microscopically examined for cancer cells).

flow cytometry—a new way of assessing cancer cells by measuring the amount of DNA (genetic material) in each cell.

flow rate (of urine)—the measurement of urine as it is expelled from the bladder. It can indicate an obstruction.

frequency (in urination)—the desire to urinate at short intervals.

gamma rays—a type of radiation like X rays but with much greater penetration. Gamma rays may be used in the treatment of prostate cancer.

general practitioner (G.P.)—a doctor who treats a wide variety of ailments. When indicated, the G.P. will refer a patient to a specialist.

gland—a group of cells which secrete certain fluids which they do not need. The fluid either goes to other parts of the body or is excreted from the body.

Gleason grading system—a way of describing prostate cancer based on the appearance of the cancer cells and their degree of differentiation. (The more differentiated, the more the cell is like a normal prostate cell and the less aggressive [fast growing] it is.)

grading—in cancer, a way to describe how malignant or aggressive a tumor is based on the microscopic appearance of the cancer cells.

gynecomastia—enlargement of a man's breasts. This can be a result of hormonal therapy.

hematospermia (hemospermia)—a slight bleeding with ejaculation. This can be a symptom of prostatitis.

hematuria—blood in the urine. When the blood is visible it is called gross hematuria. When the blood can only be seen through microscopic examination it is called microhematuria.

hesitancy (in urination)—a delayed start of the flow of urine from the body.

hormonal therapy—a form of treatment based on evidence that certain cancers depend on hormones to grow.

implant—a small container of radioactive material placed in or near a cancer. *See* INTERNAL RADIATION.

impotence (erectile dysfunction)—the inability to have an erection. An infrequent side effect of some treatments for problems of the prostate.

incontinence—the inability to hold urine in the bladder to control urination.

infection—an invasion of harmful microorganisms such as bacteria, viruses, chlamydia, or fungi into the body. Pus may be seen.

inflammation—reaction of tissue to injury; infection or irritation. The area that is affected may become painful, swollen, red, and hot.

intermittency (in urination)—a stopping and starting of the urinary stream; an inability to complete urination and empty the bladder without stopping.

internal radiation—insertion of a radioactive substance into the body in or nearby the cancer site to destroy it.

internist—a doctor who specializes in internal medicine.

interstitial radiation therapy (interstitial implant; needle implant)—a treatment in which tiny bits of radioactive isotopes inserted in hollow steel needles are implanted in and around cancerous tissue in the body. It is one type of internal radiation therapy.

intravenous pyelogram (IVP) (intravenous urogram [IVU]; excretory urogram; KUB [kidneys, ureters, bladder])—X rays taken of the urinary system (kidneys, ureters, and bladder) after the injection of a contrast dye.

kidney scan (renal scan)—an X ray examination of the structure of the kidneys after administration of a small, virtually harmless dose of a radioactive substance. A two-dimensional picture is obtained.

lateral lobes (of the prostate)—two rounded divisions of the prostate which often grow into the prostatic urethra and cause the symptoms of benign prostatic hypertrophy.

lecithin granules—small particles found in secretions of the prostate gland. When there is an infection in the prostate (prostatitis) the number of lecithin granules is decreased.

lesion—a wound, injury, or tumor.

Leydig cells—the cells in the testis that produce testosterone.

LHRH agonist—compound that is similar to a luteinizing hormone-releasing hormone. Lupron and Zoladex are two LHRH agonists which may be used in the treatment of prostate cancer. They block the production of male hormones.

libido—sexual energy and desire.

linear accelerator (megavoltage [MeV] linear accelerator; linac)—the newest machine being used in external radiation therapy. It creates high-energy radiation using electricity to form a stream of fast-moving subatomic particles. It can direct the radiation to a specific site with the least amount of damage to nearby tissue.

lobes (of the prostate)—the prostate has five distinct lobes: two lateral, a median or middle, an anterior, and a posterior.

The two lateral lobes and middle lobe are a factor in benign prostatic hypertrophy.

luteinizing hormone—a substance secreted by the pituitary gland that stimulates the secretion of sex hormones in men and women.

luteinizing hormone-releasing hormone (LHRH) (gonadotropin-releasing hormone)—a substance secreted by the brain that stimulates and controls the production of the luteinizing hormones (sex hormones) produced by the pituitary gland in both men and women.

lymph nodes—small bean-shaped structures scattered throughout the body along the channels of the lymphatic system. They filter bacteria or cancer cells that may travel through the lymphatic system.

lymphatic system—the lymph nodes, bone marrow, spleen, and thymus—which produce and store infection-fighting cells—and the network of channels that carry lymph fluid.

magnetic resonance imaging (MRI)—a highly sophisticated technique in which internal pictures of the body are produced by powerful electromagnets, radio frequency waves, and a computer. MRI does not use radiation.

male hormones—substances in the body which produce masculine characteristics. Androsterone and testosterone are the two major male hormones.

male reproductive system—that part of a man's body concerned with the production, maturation, and transportation of sperm to outside of the body.

malignant—poisonous, life-threatening. When used in a medical setting it means "cancerous."

median or middle lobe (of prostate)—one of the five lobes of the prostate. The median lobe cannot be felt during a digital rectal exam. Its enlargement is most commonly the cause of the symptoms (urination difficulty) of benign prostatic hypertrophy.

medical oncologist—a doctor who specializes in using drugs (chemotherapy) to treat cancer.

membrane—the thin layer of tissue covering or dividing an organ.

metastasis—the spread of cancer from one part of the body to another. Cells in the metastatic tumor (the second tumor) are the same as those in the original tumor. When prostate cancer metastasizes it most commonly spreads to the bone.

midstream urine (second-glass urine)—the middle part of the flow of urine (the fluid waste excreted by the kidney) collected for analysis. It is obtained in the following way: The person starts urinating, stops, and then continues into a container, then stops again and finishes urinating in a receptacle other than the container. The middle portion contains urine from the bladder, ureter, or the kidney but not from the urethra or neck of the bladder.

needle aspiration (of the prostate)—removal of a small piece of tissue from a suspicious mass in the prostate by suction with a hypodermic needle and syringe.

nocturia—a sudden sense of urgency to urinate which occurs while you are sleeping and wakes you.

nonbacterial prostatitis (noninfectious prostatitis)—inflammation of the prostate gland which is not caused by bacteria.

oncologist—a doctor who specializes in the diagnosis and treatment of cancer. There are medical, surgical, radiation, and pediatric oncologists.

orchiectomy—surgical removal of one or both testicles. The removal of both testicles leaves a man sterile and usually results in impotence and a loss of libido.

palliative therapy—a treatment not intended to cure but rather to relieve symptoms.

palpation (of the prostate)—the process of examining the prostate for abnormalities with the tip of the finger. This is done during a digital rectal exam.

pathologist—a doctor who specializes in the diagnosis of disease by studying cells and tissue removed from the body. A pathologist microscopically examines tissue to determine if cancer cells are present, what type they are, their rate of reproduction, and whether they are hormone-dependent (stimulated by hormones).

peak urine flow rate—the maximum rate of flow of urine that a person can generate. It is measured in millimeters per second.

pelvic node dissection—removal of lymph nodes near the prostate to see if they contain cancerous cells. This may be done in the diagnosis and evaluation of prostate cancer.

penile prosthesis or implant—a synthetic material surgically inserted into the penis of an impotent man so that the penis can be sufficiently erect to penetrate the vagina.

perineal—the area of the body between the scrotum and anus.

perineal prostatectomy—surgical removal of the prostate by cutting into the space between the scrotum and the anus, which is called the perineum.

perineal surgery (perineal radical prostatectomy)—an operation to remove the prostate gland through an incision made between the scrotum and anus.

pituitary gland—a small organ located at the base of the brain. The pituitary gland produces a variety of hormones that stimulate the release of hormones by other glands, including the testicles.

primary care physician—the doctor to whom the patient regularly goes for basic medical care. The primary care physician will refer a patient to a doctor who specializes in a specific area, such as a urologist, when necessary.

primary sex gland—a gland which is essential to reproduction, such as the testicles and penis. They are primary sexual structures because the testicles make the sperm that fertilize the egg in the woman and the penis delivers the sperm to the woman's body.

prostate—a male sex gland located just below the bladder and in front of the rectum. It produces semen, which carries sperm out of the body during ejaculation.

prostate cancer—the presence of malignant cells or a malignant tumor in the prostate.

prostate-specific antigen (PSA)—a protein in the blood that is manufactured only by the prostate.

prostate-specific antigen (PSA) test—analysis of blood for the presence of a specific protein that is only produced by the prostate. Elevated levels may be an indication of several different disorders of the prostate, including benign prostatic hypertrophy or prostate cancer.

prostatectomy—*see* RADICAL PROSTATECTOMY.

prostatic acid phosphatase (PAP)—an enzyme produced by the prostate that is elevated in some men diagnosed with prostate cancer or men whose cancer is spreading. It is not a very reliable screening device.

prostatic acid phosphatase (PAP) test—analysis of blood for the presence of a specific enzyme that is only produced by the prostate. Elevated levels may be an indication of several different disorders of the prostate, including benign prostatic hypertrophy or prostate cancer.

prostatic massage (prostatic stripping)—massaging the prostate gland in order to obtain its secretions for examination.

prostatic secretions—fluid produced in the prostate gland. It can be obtained by massaging the prostate.

prostatitis—inflammation of the prostate gland. There are five conditions that fall under this term: acute bacterial prostatitis, chronic bacterial prostatitis, nonbacterial prostatitis, prostatodynia and prostatosis.

prostatodynia (prostatalgia)—a condition in which pain is experienced in the prostate although there appears to be no cause for the pain in an examination and lab tests.

prostatosis—congestion of fluid in the prostate. More fluid is produced than is ejaculated.

prosthesis—an artificial replacement for a missing or damaged body part.

proteinuria—the presence of protein in the urine. A high level of protein in the urine can indicate an abnormal condition. This can be a sign of a damaged or diseased kidney.

pyuria—the presence of pus (white blood cells) in the urine which makes it cloudy. This can be a sign of an infection in the urinary tract.

radiation oncologist—a doctor who specializes in using radiation to treat cancer.

radiation therapy—the use of high-energy waves or particles to treat disease. Radiation therapy can be administered from outside the body by a machine, or inside the body by implanting radioactive materials into or near the targeted site.

radical prostatectomy—surgical removal of the prostate and the tissue around it, including the capsule and seminal vesicles.

radiologist—a physician who specializes in reading diagnostic X rays and performing specialized X-ray procedures.

rectoscope (proctoscope)—a thin, lighted instrument about six inches long used in transurethral resection.

rectum—the last five or six inches of the colon leading to the outside of the body.

renal scan—*see* KIDNEY SCAN.

residual urine—urine that remains in the bladder after voiding. Any amount is considered abnormal.

retrograde ejaculation—during male orgasm sperm shoots back into the bladder instead of exiting through the penis. This can be a side effect of prostate surgery.

retropubic prostatectomy—surgical removal of the prostate through an incision in the abdomen.

scrotum—the external pouch or sac which contains the testes and their accessory organs.

second-glass urine—*see* MIDSTREAM URINE.

semen—a thick, whitish fluid produced by the prostate. Sperm are carried by semen.

seminal vesicles—a pair of small sacs located just behind the bladder. Seminal vesicles provide nutrients for sperm and may store sperm as well.

simulation—a process in which X-ray pictures are used to plan radiation treatment so that the area to be treated is precisely located and marked for treatment.

sitz bath—a tub in which a person can sit with enough water to cover the perineum (the space between the anus and scrotum). Soaking in warm to hot water to which various bath salts have been added can relieve pain or discomfort in the perineal area.

sperm—mature germ cells produced by the testicles which can fertilize the ova (egg cells) in a woman.

sperm banking—the freezing and storing of a man's sperm (male fertilizing cells) so that they can be used in the future for procreation if the man becomes infertile.

sphincter—a ringlike band of muscle fibers that can constrict a passage or close an opening in the body. By contracting the urinary sphincter a man can shut off his urinary system (stop urinating).

stage—in cancer, the tumor size and extent of spread of disease.

staging—an evaluation of the patient, after a diagnosis of cancer, to find out where else the cancer might be. Every case of cancer must be staged in order to determine the correct treatment.

stress incontinence—the inability to control urination when there is sudden intra-abdominal pressure from something like a sneeze or cough.

stricture (of the urethra)—a narrowing of the urethra as a result of the growth of abnormal tissue or scarring. This can result in difficulty in urination.

surgery—the treatment of disease by removal of tissue, usually by some kind of cutting device. It is the oldest and still most common treatment for cancer and the most common treatment of benign prostatic hypertrophy.

testicles (testes)—the two egg-shaped glands located directly under the penis. Sperm (male reproductive cells) are formed in the testicles.

testosterone—a male sex hormone produced chiefly by the

testicles. Testosterone stimulates a man's sexual activity as well as the growth of other sex organs, including the prostate.

three-glass urine—a particular way of collecting urine used in the diagnosis of prostatitis. Three samples of urine are collected along with a sample of prostate fluid.

third-glass urine—the urine that is collected after prostatic stripping (massage).

tissue—a group of cells organized to perform a specific function.

transabdominal ultrasound—a procedure which may be used in the diagnosis and/or evaluation of benign prostatic hypertrophy and prostate cancer. A special device is moved over the abdomen to produce ultrasound pictures of the prostate.

transrectal fine-needle aspiration biopsy (needle biopsy, fine-needle aspiration MRI [FNA]-or fine-needle biopsy)—a special needle which contains a minuscule cutting instrument is used in the removal of tissue in order to perform microscopic examination for cancer cells.

transrectal ultrasound (TRUS)—a procedure which may be used in the diagnosis and evaluation of benign prostatic hypertrophy and prostate cancer. A probe is inserted in the rectum and an ultrasound is taken.

transurethral—the route through the urethra.

transurethral incision of the prostate (TUIP)—a fairly new surgical procedure used in the treatment of an enlarged prostate. A resectoscope cuts and splits the prostate to relieve pressure on the urethra, thereby restoring normal urinary functioning.

transurethral resection of the prostate (TUR or TURP)—The use of a special instrument inserted through the penis to remove a small benign or malignant prostate tumor.

tumor—an abnormal tissue growth in or on the body that serves no useful purpose. Tumors can be benign (noncancerous) or malignant (cancerous).

tumor marker—a substance found in increased amounts in the body fluids of some cancer patients.

tumor-nodes-metastases (TNM)—a system used in the staging of cancer. The *T* stands for tumor, the *N* stands for lymph node involvement and the *M* stands for metastases. A number following the letter indicates the size of the tumor, the extent of lymph node involvement and the extent of metastatic disease.

ultrasound (sonogram; ultrasonography)—a diagnostic procedure that bounces high-frequency sound waves off tissues and changes the echoes into pictures. Ultrasound can be used to find and measure solid tumors in the body.

uremia—poisoning from urine substances in the blood.

ureter—the tube that carries urine from each kidney to the bladder.

urethra—the tube that carries urine from the bladder and semen from the prostate to the outside of the body.

urologist—a doctor who specializes in diseases of the urinary organs in females and the urinary and sex organs in men.

X ray—high-energy radiation that at low levels can be used in the diagnosis of cancer and at high levels can be used to treat it.